The Essential Plant-Based Pantry

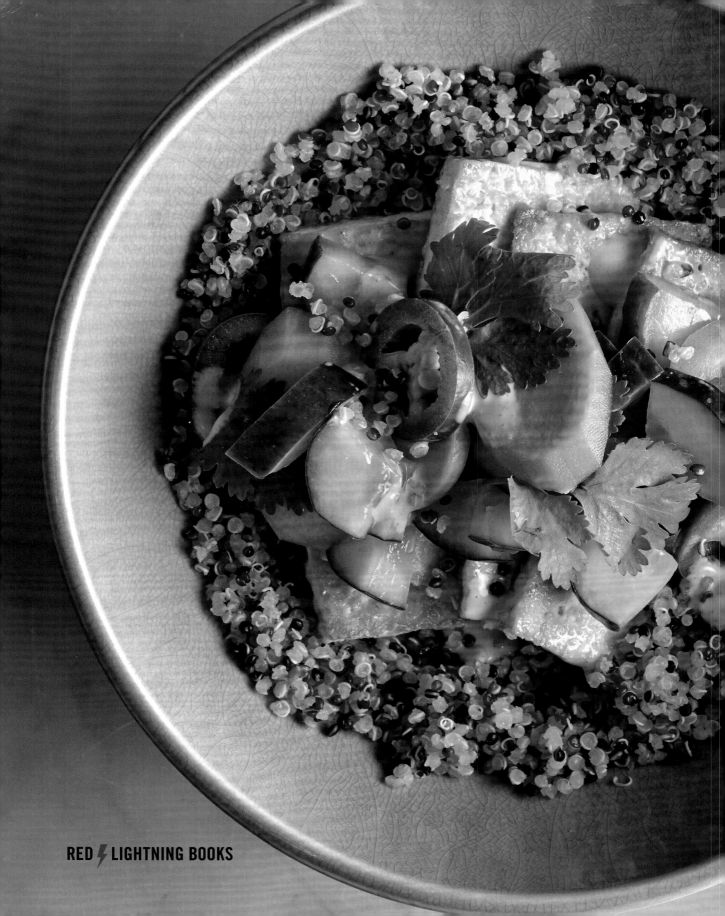

RED ⚡ LIGHTNING BOOKS

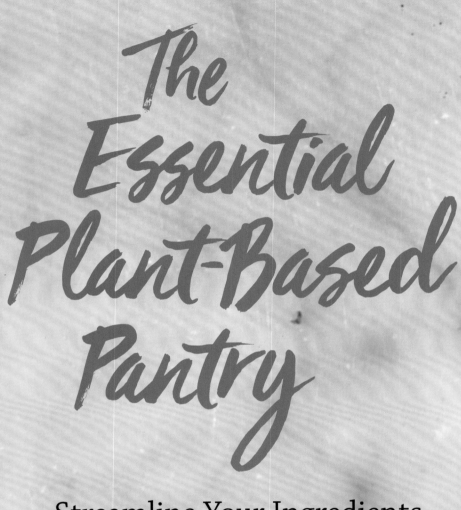

The Essential Plant-Based Pantry

Streamline Your Ingredients, Simplify Your Meals

Maggie Green

Photographs by Sarah Jane Sanders

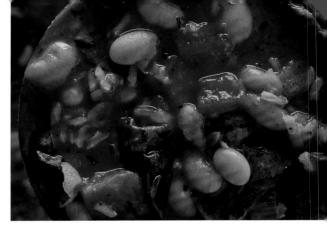

This book is a publication of

Red Lightning Books
1320 East 10th Street
Bloomington, Indiana 47405 USA

redlightningbooks.com

© 2018 by Maggie Green,
Photographs by Sarah Jane Sanders

All rights reserved

No part of this book may be reproduced or
utilized in any form or by any means,
electronic or mechanical, including photocopy-
ing and recording, or by any information storage
and retrieval system, without permission in
writing from the publisher. The paper used in
this publication meets the minimum require-
ments of the American National Standard for
Information Sciences—Permanence of Paper for
Printed Library Materials, ANSI z39.48-1992.

Manufactured in China

ISBN: 978-1-68435-010-0 <cloth>
ISBN: 978-1-68435-046-9 <ebook>

1 2 3 4 5 22 21 20 19 18

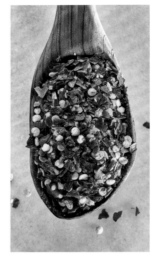

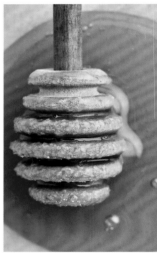

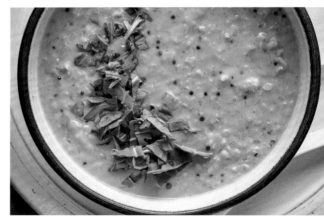

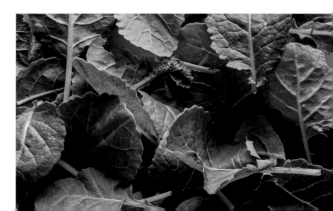

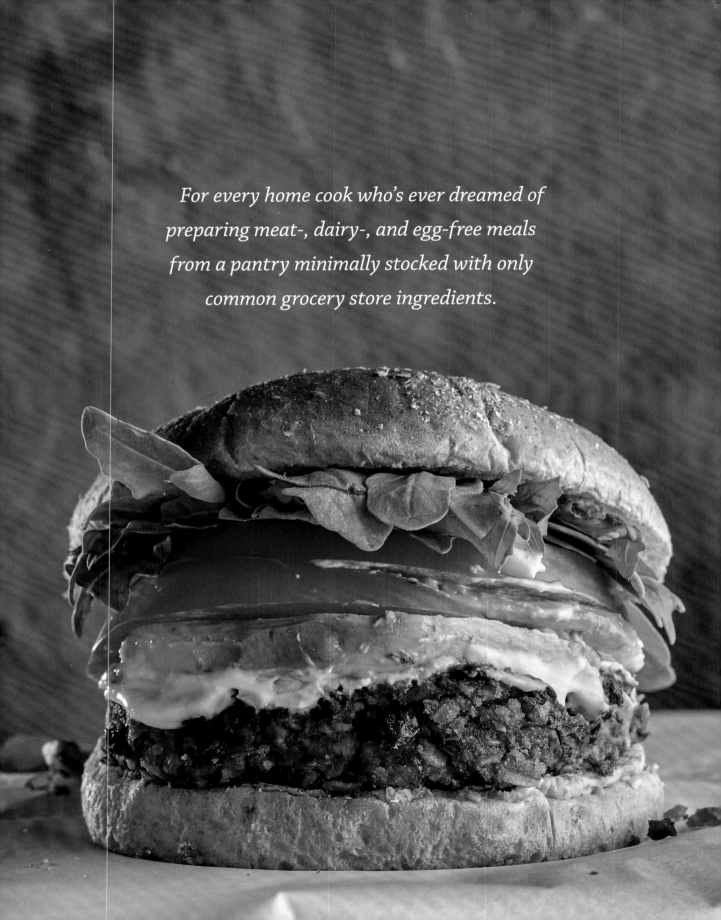

For every home cook who's ever dreamed of preparing meat-, dairy-, and egg-free meals from a pantry minimally stocked with only common grocery store ingredients.

Contents

Sips and Small Plates

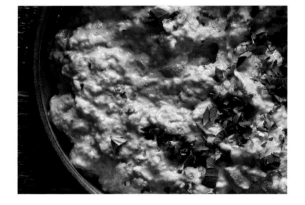

Sauces

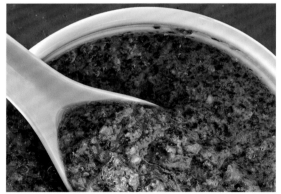

Soups   60

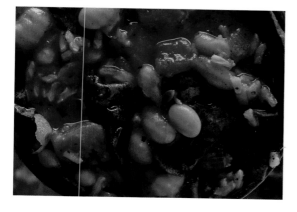

Salads   76

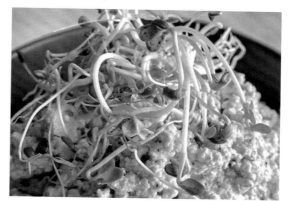

Sides   102

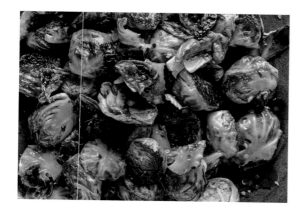

Suppers and Savory Bowls   120

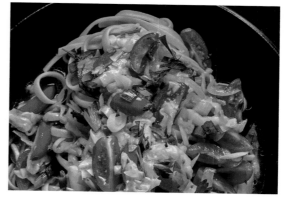

Acknowledgments

Writing one cookbook manuscript takes time, patience, and focus. Writing two manuscripts at the same time was a test of my organizational skills and my ability to compartmentalize my mind, something I'm used to doing in my "day job," but not anything I've done with writing cookbooks. I initially wasn't asked to submit the manuscripts for this book and *The Essential Pantry* together, but the fact that I made the decision to, and followed through on that plan, feels satisfying. Now I know that cooks can use either, or both, of the *Essential Pantry* books to create over one hundred recipes for tasty meat- and plant-based food with a very similar core set of pantry ingredients.

As with all cookbooks I've written, this wasn't a solitary project. I provide the guts of the book, and many people helped along the way.

The leading main man and the best male cook I know, Warren Green continues to stand beside me at all times. His attention to detail is unmatched by anyone I've ever met. This comes in handy for recipe development, where he tastes, smells, and critiques; in food preparation, when he's always willing to shop for ingredients or wash the dishes; and when it's time to read recipes and manuscripts and his sharp eye and even-sharper pencil make my work better. For this, and for his expanding hobby of brewing ales and lagers, I am forever grateful.

At the heart of what I do, our three children, Stuart, Julia, and Neil, have grown up with me in the kitchen tinkering with my own recipes, or with recipes for a project or client. No matter what's going on, they are always willing to taste the fruits of my labor and provide their feedback, even when the food was meat, egg, and dairy free. They now have friends who join the tasting sessions, and that is a lot of fun. I never imagined that when my teens left our home for high school, college, co-ops, fraternity life, and time with other families and friends, my heart would continue to grow in love and appreciation for them, their hard work, and what they bring to our family as their horizons expand beyond our kitchen table. For this book, I especially want to thank my sweet daughter, Julia. Her exploration of plant-based eating was the impetus for this book. Our experiment with no meat, dairy, or eggs lasted almost one year. We had fun together exploring this way of eating and cooking. If you choose to eat this way, I know the kitchen is a place you're familiar with.

A proud member of the *Essential Plant-Based Pantry* team, professional photographer Sarah Jane Sanders is a true joy to work with. I've had the benefit of working with Sarah Jane more than once, and for that I am appreciative. Sarah sees food and ingredients through the lens of a camera in a way that not many photographers do. I thank her for her expertise to bring the concept of common pantry ingredients, and recipes from these ingredients, to life for this book.

In touch and always helpful, my acquisitions editor, Ashley Runyon, contacted me and asked me to submit my idea for this cookbook, and its companion book, *The Essential Pantry*. Ashley was always available to answer questions, give her opinion, and provide whatever I needed while I wrote the manuscripts. I thank her for her confidence in me, my ideas, and my ability to write two cookbooks at one time.

On my mind are the individuals who dedicated their time, ingredients, and utilities to the recipe-testing portion of the *Essential Plant-Based Pantry* project. The dedicated and willing testers for this book all responded to my request for recipes testers, and when I asked if they could do more, I was generally in receipt of an enthusiastic yes. I know that their work helped shape these recipes into formulas that cooks everywhere can use to achieve good-tasting results: Robert Anderson, Mary Anderson, Frances Banks, Kyle Baumann, Lori Bright, Suzanne Caithamer, Heather Chapman, Alex Flamm, Elizabeth Flamm, Kaye Flamm, Patty Grasty, Warren Green, Julia Green, Carl Kroboth, Brandy Mohktar, Lori Moser, Gwen McCormack, Luisa Polito, Mejie Renaud, Sharon Thompson, and Tammy Yancey.

Working behind the scenes to edit, design, print, market, and sell this book was Red Lightning Press. I thank all who took my manuscript and turned it into a finished book, including my editor, Rachel Rosolina, and my designer, Pamela Rude.

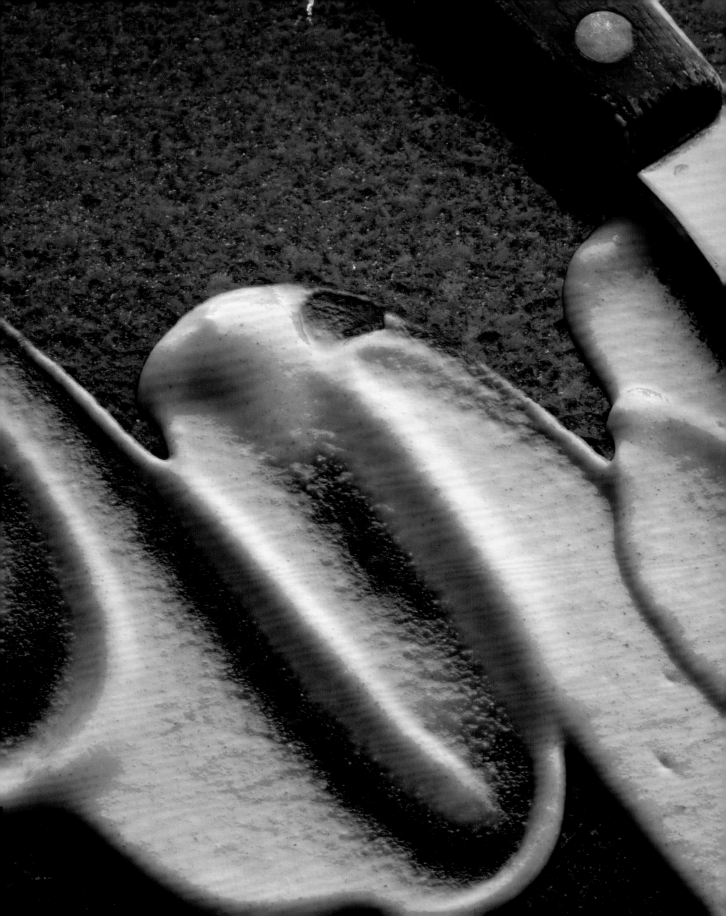

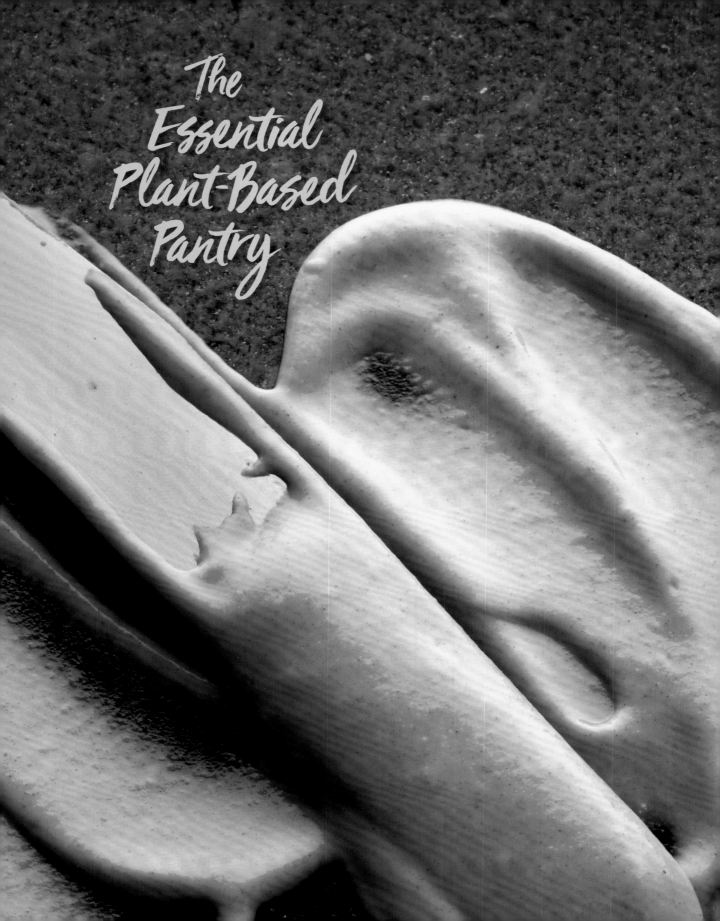

The
Essential
Plant-Based
Pantry

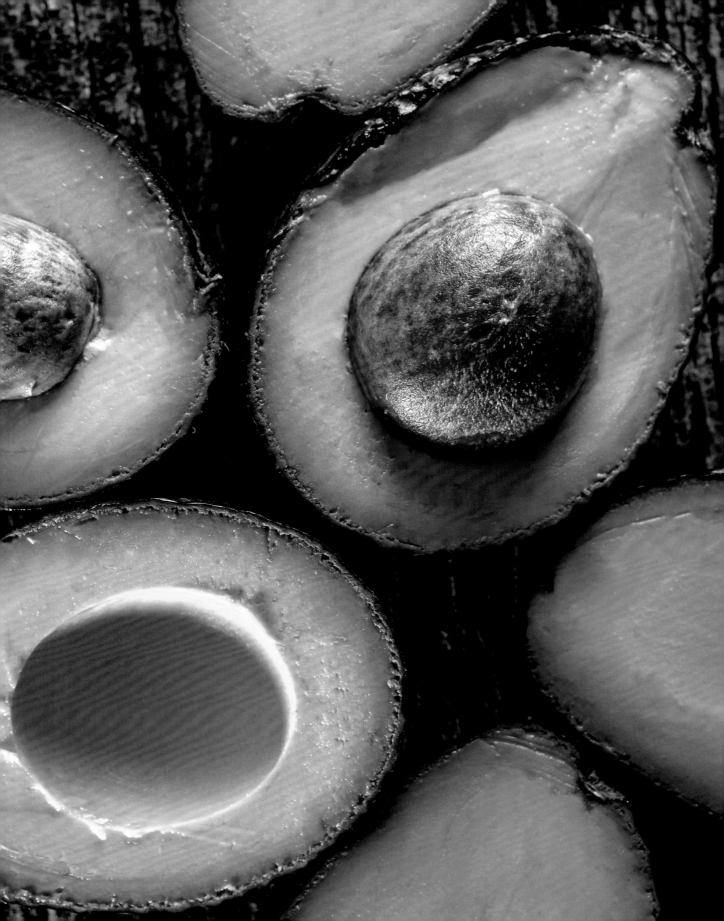

Introduction

My first cookbook, *The Kentucky Fresh Cookbook*, was an offshoot of my personal chef business. That book contained recipes I had grown to love and that I cooked for clients and at home. Prior to writing that book, I kept track of everything I cooked for my family's evening meals for two years. When I studied these notes, I noticed a seasonality to what I cooked. Meals changed based on the time of the year. The weather changed, what's in season changed, and holidays came and went. The result was a book connected to seasonal cooking in Kentucky with twelve month-by-month chapters.

Despite my success with *The Kentucky Fresh Cookbook*, I began to notice how infrequently I turned to recipes when I cooked everyday food and meals. Without ever referencing a cookbook or printed recipes, I can create a menu for the week, write a grocery list based on what I plan to cook, and shop for ingredients. As a result, I have everything I need in my pantry, refrigerator, and freezer for the next week's meals. This is my sweet spot and a system I've used for over twenty years.

To those outside of my immediate family, this seemed fascinating. So, I began to study how I managed to pull off this meal preparation routine year in and year out. The answer was right in front of me—a stocked pantry and the knowledge that I had basic ingredients on hand for the meals I wanted to cook. I simply had to buy the fresh ingredients and restock any ingredients I ran out of the previous week. And then, when my teenage daughter decided she wanted to eat more plant-based meals, and explore vegan recipes, my stocked pantry became an even more important source of plant-based ingredients. Canned beans, canned tomatoes, and coconut milk. Rice, grains, and pasta. Dried thyme, basil, and curry powder. Tahini, sesame oil, and quinoa. All are common ingredients found in a supermarket, and all are in my pantry, ready to be used when I cook those recipes in my head—especially during my plant-based journey with my daughter.

I've spent a large part of my professional career with my nose in cookbooks and recipes. If I wasn't being paid to read a cookbook or develop and test recipes, I was using my time to develop and test my own recipes, and write my own books. As a trained chef, former food service director, cookbook editor, author, home cook, cookbook lover, and cookbook coach, I still spend a large part of my day with recipes and cookbooks. So, it comes as no surprise to me that most cooks are driven by recipes. In our bookstores and online, we are inundated with recipes. We have binders full of recipes for inspiration, social media folders and boards full of recipe ideas, and shelves full of cookbooks.

But, here's the catch—when it's time to prepare the recipes, we don't have the ingredients in our pantries for the recipes we want to cook. I'd argue that recipes aren't the problem. We have an abundance of them. Maybe the problem is our planning. Perhaps it feels overwhelming to shop for everything. I also speculate that the problem is our pantry. It doesn't store what we need in order to cook the recipes we want to cook. On top of that, some recipes may require that we shop at more than one store to find everything we need. Then when we do shop, we may buy ingredients we never use again. They sit in our pantries, unused, and taking up space. So what do we do? We throw in the towel, chuck the recipes, forget the pantry, and head to a drive-through for dinner. Or we resort to food assembly with premade sauces, salads, and entrees, because they're easy and predictable. Who cares if we eat the same thing all the time?

Up to this point, even my own cookbooks haven't offered a solution. They certainly supply recipes, but they also require scattered shopping at more than one location to find ingredients, as well as one-time-use ingredients.

I decided it was time to put my money where my mouth is. I decided it was time to write a cookbook using *only* a core set of plant-based pantry ingredients. I imagined this to be a challenge, sort of like music, which uses only eight notes (plus sharps and flats) to create such a variety of beautiful melodies, and sort of like the English language, with an alphabet of twenty-six letters and well over 170,000 words (according to the second edition of *The Oxford English Dictionary*). If I used approximately fifty pantry ingredients, how many recipes could I create? *The Essential Plant-Based Pantry* is the result of my experiment.

The Essential Plant-Based Pantry can change the way you shop and cook plant-based meals. It may even change the way you think about cooking foods that are meat, dairy, and egg free. When you realize how easy this concept is, that all you have to do is stock your pantry and know you have everything you need, the light will go on, and so will the oven. *The Essential Plant-Based Pantry* gets you out of the suppertime rut where we read recipes, buy cookbooks, and think about cooking, but opt for fast-food instead. *The Essential Plant-Based Pantry* puts meals within reach because you now have everything you need—with a pantry that serves you. With this book you now have the recipes *and* the stocked pantry. All you have to do is buy the fresh ingredients!

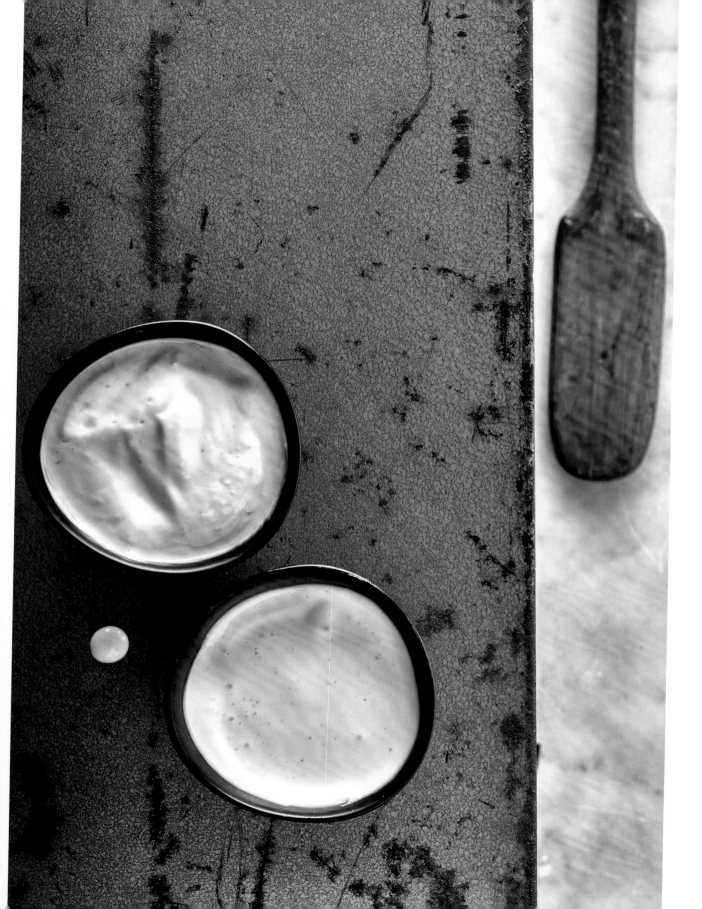

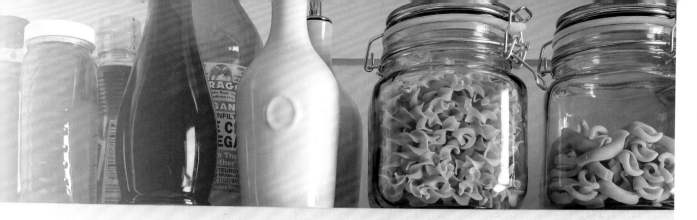
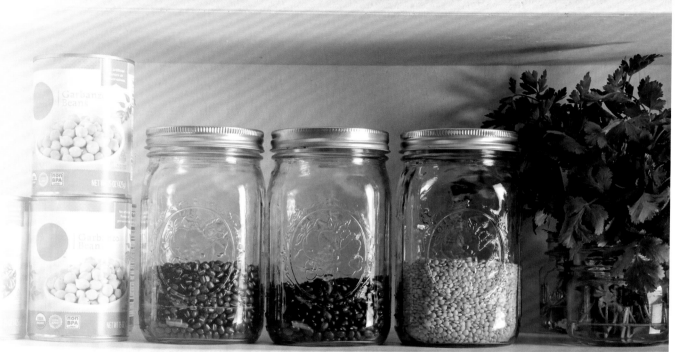
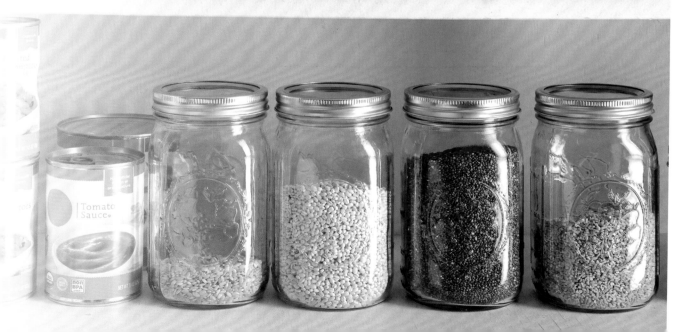

The Essential Plant-Based Pantry Concept

Here's what you get with *The Essential Plant-Based Pantry:*

A list—With *The Essential Plant-Based Pantry* ingredient list, page 6, you can stock your pantry ahead of time. This list contains dry goods, some refrigerated items, and a few frozen foods.

A set of recipes—*The Essential Plant-Based Pantry* contains over sixty recipes that use only *Essential Plant-Based Pantry* ingredients.

A guarantee—The ingredients listed in this book can be purchased at a well-stocked supermarket, and all ingredients are used more than once.

A promise—All you do is buy the fresh ingredients and restock the dry goods as you use them.

A change in attitude—*The Essential Plant-Based Pantry* just might change the way you think and feel about cooking when you realize that you already have everything you need in order to cook a meal.

Why should you invest in *The Essential Plant-Based Pantry* concept? Or in this book? Let's just say that with this book you can make your pantry smaller and more efficient. With this book, you can create recipes knowing that you have the ingredients in your pantry. And, you need this book if you are a home cook or organizing buff who wants to:

- Prepare more meat-, egg-, and dairy-free meals at home
- Select from your choice of gluten-free recipes as well
- Find what you need in one trip to the supermarket
- Avoid multiple trips to specialty stores to shop for ingredients you only use once
- Avoid subscribing to a meal-kit service
- Overhaul your cluttered pantry
- Create a well-organized pantry with useful ingredients
- Prepare meals with real ingredients
- Stock the pantry in your boat, condo, RV, travel trailer, or tiny house with limited ingredients

The Essential Plant-Based Pantry Ingredient List

Who doesn't love a stocked pantry, a designated area in your kitchen filled with ingredients for meal preparation? Officially defined as a small room or closet in which food, dishes, or utensils are kept, pantries are popular in kitchens of all sizes. Kitchen designers report that a pantry is almost always a consideration in kitchen design because everyone wants a place to store dry goods. But what they really want is a pantry that serves them, where they know they have on hand the dry goods they need to cook.

This plant-based ingredient list contains everything you need to make every recipe in this book. Some ingredients are used more than others, and in some ways, I feel like I've just scratched the recipes that can be created with these ingredients. Consider this book a good place to start, and then let our imagination guide the rest of the journey with your pantry.

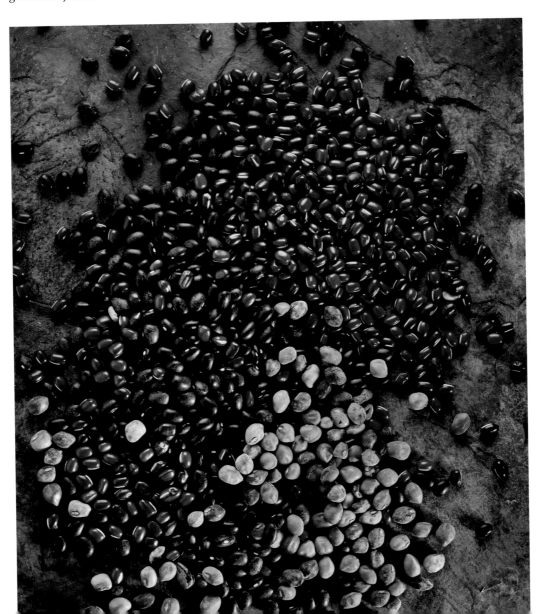

Dry Herbs and Spices

basil, dried
cardamom, ground
cayenne pepper
chili powder
cinnamon, ground
coriander, ground
cumin, ground
curry powder
dill weed, dried
garlic powder
ginger, powdered
onion powder
oregano, dried
pepper, black peppercorns for
    grinding
red pepper flakes
salt, kosher
smoked paprika
thyme, dried
turmeric, ground

Dry Goods

beans, dry black, chickpeas, kidney, red,
    great northern (if not using canned)
barley, pearl
cocoa powder, unsweetened
cranberries, dried
flour, all-purpose
lentils, brown
lentils, red
nuts, raw cashews
nuts, sliced almonds
nuts, walnuts
oats, old-fashioned
pasta, spaghetti, linguine,
    fettuccine, rotini, penne
quinoa
raisins, golden
rice, basmati
rice, brown
seeds, pumpkin
sugar, light brown
sugar, white
wheat berries

Canned or Bottled Foods

beans, black beans
beans, chickpeas
beans, kidney
beans, red beans
beans, great northern
broth, vegetable
capers
chipotle in adobo
chiles, green chopped
coconut milk
honey
hot sauce, Frank's RedHot
mustard, Dijon
oil, canola or other vegetable oil
oil, olive
oil, toasted sesame
olives, green pitted
olives, Kalamata pitted
peanut butter
red peppers, roasted
sriracha
tahini
tamari or reduced-sodium soy sauce
tomato paste
tomato sauce
tomatoes, crushed
tomatoes, diced fire-roasted
vinegar, apple cider
vinegar, red wine
wine, red

Nondairy Refrigerated

milk, almond or cashew
tofu, extra-firm
tofu, silken
tempeh

Frozen

edamame, shelled
corn, frozen

The Essential Plant-Based Pantry Makover

1. Familiarize yourself with *The Essential Pantry* ingredient list, page 6.
2. Start fresh with a pantry overhaul.
   a. Empty your pantry of everything.
   b. Throw away old spices and herbs.
   c. Wipe off the shelving.
   d. Vacuum the floor and the corners.
   e. Compare what you have to *The Essential Plant-Based Pantry* ingredient list.
   f. Mark any ingredients you need to buy.
   g. Buy any dry goods you need.
   h. Restock your *Essential Plant-Based Pantry* ingredients.
3. Post *The Essential Plant-Based Pantry* ingredient list on your refrigerator.
4. Plan your week and identify the recipe(s) you want to make.
5. Buy the fresh produce.
6. Prepare the recipes as planned.
7. Note on *The Essential Plant-Based Pantry* ingredient list any dry goods you're out of or low on.
8. Buy pantry items the next time you buy the fresh items to keep your pantry stocked and ready to roll.

The Essential Plant-Based Pantry Menus

I think it's nice to provide combinations of food for meals, so here's my best shot at giving you some suggestions. I also make menu suggestions in the recipe's headnotes, so be sure to read the recipe introductions for more ideas.

Fettuccine Cashew Alfredo
Sesame Honey Brussels Sprouts

Fried Tofu
Tomato Curry Sauce
Mediterranean Salad

Moroccan Tempeh
Cardamom Carrots
Bean Salad with Lime Vinaigrette

Tofu Shakshuka
Cooked Wheat Berries
Apple Celery Salad

Curry Coconut Chickpeas
Spiced Rice Pilaf
Cardamom Carrots

Tomato White Bean Soup
Tofu Egg Salad Sandwiches

Pan-Roasted Tomato Sauce
Whole-Grain Penne Pasta
Baby Spinach with Fresh Herb Vinaigrette

Cashew Cream of Broccoli Soup
Sweet Spicy Chickpea Salad

Cincinnati Lentil Chili
Mediterranean Salad

Spicy Marinara Sauce
Whole-Grain Spaghetti
Spring Greens with Fresh Herb Vinaigrette

Barbecue Lentils
Napa Cabbage Slaw with Sriracha
    Peanut Sauce
Mac and No Cheese
Refrigerator Pickles

Summer Linguine
Vietnamese Spring Roll Salad with Sweet
    Chile Vinaigrette

Curried Red Lentil Soup
Skillet Tofu Hash
Sriracha Plant-Based Mayonnaise
Apple and Celery Salad

Smoky Red Beans and Rice
Kale Salad

Fried Tofu
Barbecue Sauce
Napa Cabbage Slaw with Sriracha
    Peanut Sauce
Sweet Potato and Onion Hash Browns

Fried Tofu
Barbecue Sauce
Edamame Succotash
Kale Salad

Kidney Bean Burgers
Kale Salad
Mac and No Cheese

Lentil Barley Soup
Tofu Eggless Salad
Refrigerator Pickles

Vegetable Curry with Rice
Napa Cabbage Slaw with
    Sriracha Peanut Sauce

Vegetable Kale Soup
Barbecue Lentils (sandwich)
Refrigerator Pickles

Creamy Chickpea Marinara
Whole-Grain Penne or Rigatoni
Carrot Golden Raisin Salad

Using *The Essential Plant-Based Pantry* Recipes

Other than practice, a complimentary path to becoming a better cook is to pay attention to your selection of ingredients. Even with a stocked pantry, I believe that the use of some fresh herbs over dry, fresh citrus juice over bottled, fresh garlic when appropriate, freshly ground black pepper and kosher salt to taste, and the careful use of cayenne pepper or hot sauce go a long way in making a cook a better cook. Here are some tips:

- Buy the highest quality ingredients you can buy for the dollar.

- Read the recipe in its entirety before embarking on the cooking process. I sometimes bury tips and suggestions in the headnotes, so don't skip those.

- Chop and measure ingredients first, so everything is in its place before the cooking begins.

- Taste the food as the recipe proceeds. This will help you adjust salt and pepper as you go along.

- Most recipes recommend a quantity of salt and pepper to use. In the end, season food to suit your personal taste and preference, as that preference may not match my preference.

- **Salt**—In the testing of these recipes, I used kosher salt. If you use standard table salt when you cook, you should start using less salt than is called for in the recipes.

- **Fresh herbs**—When I finish dishes with herbs, I prefer to use fresh. Parsley, mint, cilantro, rosemary, and basil are fresh herbs I most commonly use. Dried versions of these herbs aren't as good as fresh for finishing. Fresh always looks prettier and tastes fresher.

- **Lemon and lime juice**—There's no doubt, fresh lemon and lime juice are my choices for all recipes. I keep lemons in the refrigerator, so I have them on hand to use in cooking. They are one simple ingredient with unlimited potential to brighten up a pot of soup, a pie filling, or fresh, homemade vinaigrette.

- **Pasta**—I use a variety of dry pasta shapes in both traditional- and whole-grain, or legume-based styles. Of course, the use of whole-grain or even gluten-free pasta is a personal choice, so any pasta of your choice should work well, including those that are based on grains other than flour.

- **Black pepper**—Freshly ground black pepper is the pepper of choice for all recipes. Season to taste, as everyone has a different tolerance for black pepper.

- **Olive oil**—I generally use a nice, store-bought olive oil to cook with and don't spend the extra dollars on a high-end extra virgin for cooking.

Gluten-Free Recipes

Recipes marked with the gluten-free tag are free of gluten-containing or possible-gluten-containing ingredients, such as pasta, bread, all-purpose flour, tamari, oats, or barley. This tag is intended to assist those who choose gluten-free meals and recipes. For those with medically diagnosed gluten sensitivity, or celiac disease, it is recommended that you follow prescribed medical nutrition therapy guidelines. Cross-contamination can occur in processing plants with ingredients that are inherently gluten-free. Use your best judgment about cross-contamination, or extreme sensitivity, as the recipes tagged "gluten-free" here are is not medical advice.

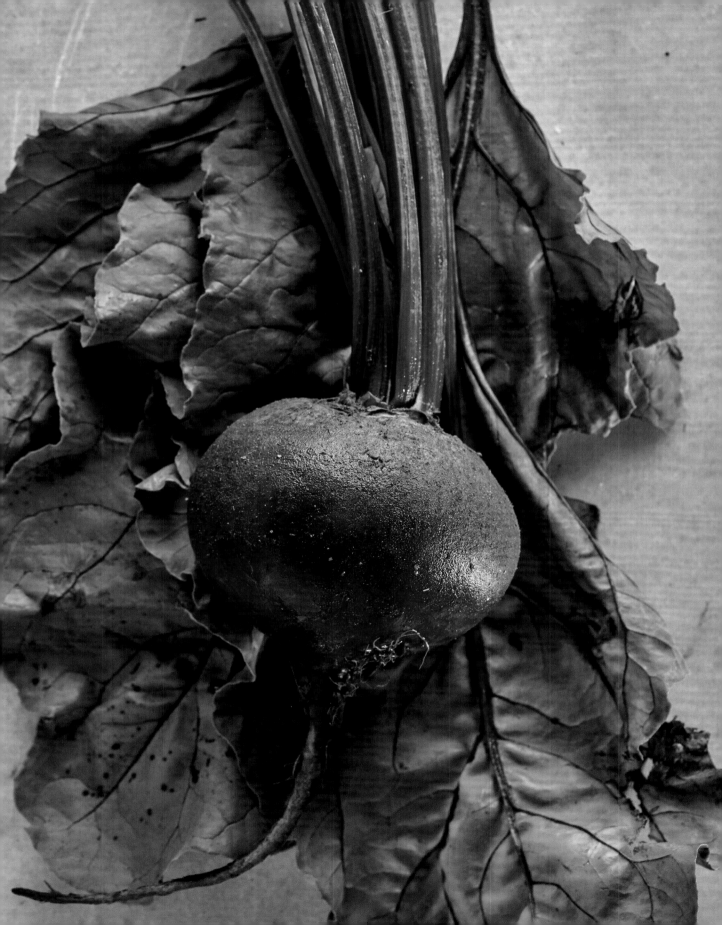

Sips and Small Plates

There are a lot of reasons to prepare a refreshing drink or a flavorful spread or dip. Whether you start the day, take a pause after school, or run out the door to a gathering, these recipes add plant-based creaminess, flavor, and spice to any occasion. The spreads are easily prepared ahead and tucked in the refrigerator. All you need is a whole-grain baguette or fresh sliced vegetables, and you're snack- or party-ready. With a smoothie or hot cup of cocoa, you can enjoy drinks that supply plant-based and pantry-ready proteins.

Recipes

Turmeric Cocoa Latte

Banana Cocoa-Nut Smoothie

Spicy Refrigerator Pickles

Buffalo Tofu

Olive Spread

Green Hummus

Roasted White Bean Dip

Smoky Eggplant Dip

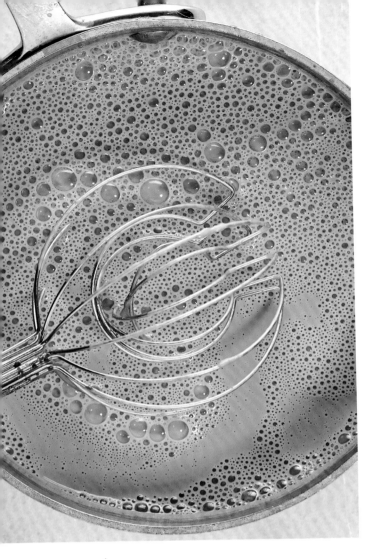

Turmeric Cocoa Latte gluten free

Serves 2

Golden Milk is a popular westernized version of traditional Indian *haldi doodh*, or turmeric milk, made with almond milk, turmeric, honey, and spices. Beejoli Shah, in an October 2016 article for *Bon Appetit*, described traditional haldi doodh as "simple: half a cup or less of piping hot milk, with a tablespoon of ground turmeric dissolved into it until the entire mixture, is a bright yellow." This recipe westernizes Golden Milk even more by combining popular pantry items—cocoa powder and turmeric—to create a beverage that brings my life-long fascination with spices together in a warm drink. Any nut milk can be used here. Alternatively, serve over ice.

Ingredients:

2 teaspoons unsweetened cocoa powder

1 teaspoon ground turmeric

½ teaspoon powdered ginger

1 tablespoon honey

1 tablespoon water

2 cups almond, cashew, soy, or beverage-style coconut milk

Freshly ground black pepper

Directions:

In a small saucepan whisk together the cocoa powder, turmeric, ginger, honey, and water to make a thin paste. Whisk in 1/4 cup of the almond milk and blend well. Whisk in the remaining almond milk. Place over medium heat and whisk occasionally until steam starts to rise from the surface and the milk just starts to bubble gently. Remove from the heat and cover the pan. Let sit for 10 minutes before serving. Whisk until bubbly and serve hot, topped with freshly ground black pepper, or allow it to cool and serve over ice.

Turmeric Powder

Ground dried turmeric powder adds bright yellow color to food along with a pungent flavor. An ancient spice touted for its anti-inflammatory properties, turmeric will stain your hands, dishcloths, and cutting boards a nice shade of yellow. Mix with water to create a yellow dye for hard-cooked eggs.

14

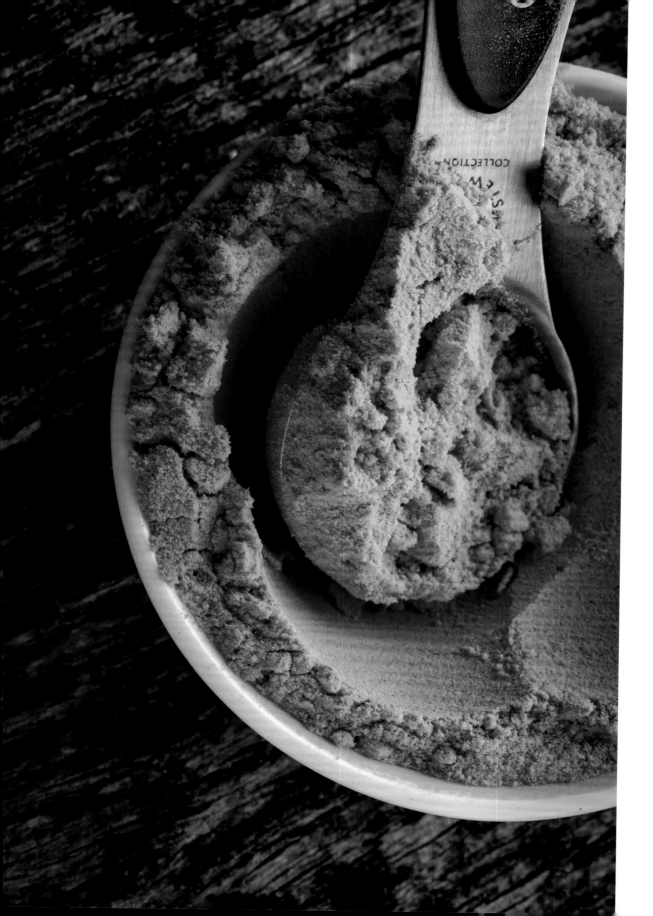

Banana Cocoa-Nut Smoothie

gluten free

Serves 2

Freeze your bananas before making this smoothie, or add crushed ice (or six ice cubes) if making this with a room-temperature banana. To freeze a banana for a smoothie, peel and slice the banana. Place the banana slices in a small zip-top bag. Flatten the bag's contents so you don't have a big clump of bananas, and freeze at least overnight. Now they are ready for a twirl in the blender.

Ingredients:

1 medium-size banana, sliced and frozen

1 ½ cups almond, soy, cashew, or beverage-style coconut milk

1 tablespoon unsweetened cocoa powder

1 tablespoon peanut butter

½ teaspoon cinnamon

Optional: ½ cup crushed ice or 6 ice cubes

Directions:

To make the smoothie, blend the sliced frozen banana, nut milk, cocoa powder, peanut butter, and cinnamon. Add optional ice if banana is not frozen. Serve in a tall glass or divide between two smaller glasses.

Coconut Milk

At the supermarket, coconut milk is sold in shelf-stable cans or boxes or as a beverage-style blend in refrigerated cartons.

If not specified in a recipe, canned coconut milk works best in soups, curries, stews, and other dishes or drinks that are heated so that the coconut fat melts and blends in to the dish or drink. It's personal preference whether you select regular or lite coconut milk. Sometimes the light coconut milk is not as flavorful because it contains less of the coconut fat.

Beverage-style coconut milk contains coconut milk with added sugar, salt, and thickeners. It is sold refrigerated and is intended for drinking and not cooking. It works well for hot or cold beverages, smoothies, or coffee.

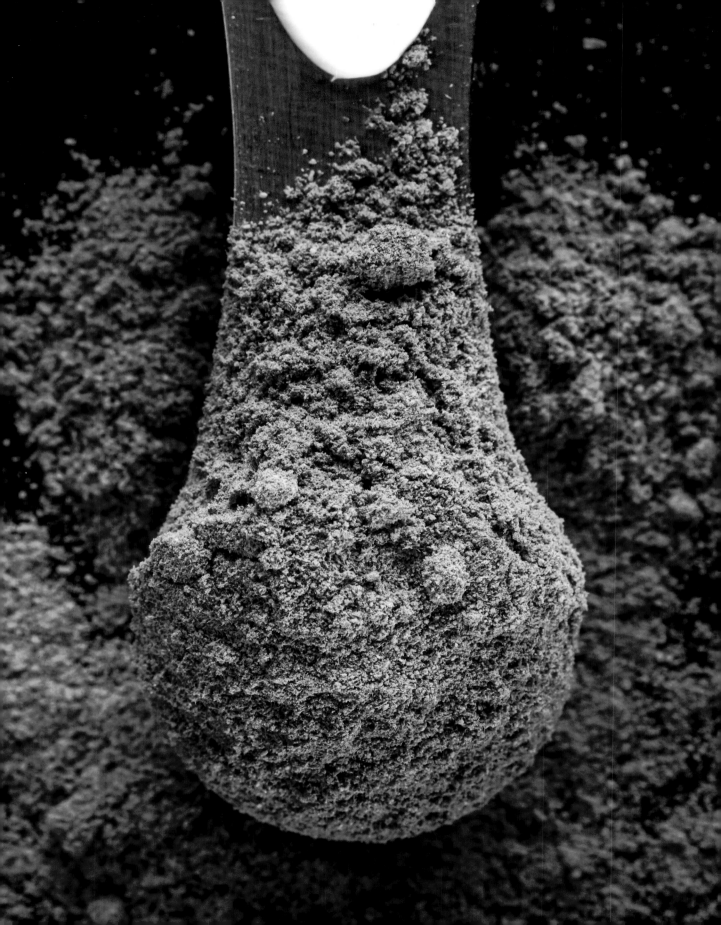

Spicy Refrigerator Pickles

gluten free

Makes 1 quart

Before you dismiss this recipe, please reconsider. I hope this changes the way you think and feel about making homemade pickles. All of the pickle brine ingredients are found in your pantry, so all you have to do is prepare four cups of vegetables and heat the brine.

You may think this recipe isn't for you or is "out of reach" if you don't have a garden, a canner, or all day to spend in the kitchen. Designed specifically with these barriers in mind, this recipe makes exactly one quart of pickled vegetables and is probably one of the easiest things you could ever make. The recipe can be easily doubled. Two suggested veggie mixes are listed below, although you can use any combination of vegetables. No matter what vegetables you use, you need four cups of prepared vegetables. Ideas other than what's listed below include zucchini spears, red pepper strips, onion chunks, or whole green beans.

Pickle vinegar brine ingredients:

½ cup apple cider vinegar

1 ¾ cup water

2 tablespoons sugar

2 tablespoons kosher salt

½ teaspoon red pepper flakes or black peppercorns (optional for the Spicy Bahn Mi Mix because it already contains jalapeño and is spicy without the pepper)

Directions:

Thoroughly wash the jar and lid. Fill the jar with boiling water and cover the lid with boiling water to sterilize. Pour out the hot water before filling.

Prepare the vegetables. If using fresh dill, put the dill sprig in the jar first. Pack the vegetables and crushed garlic in the jar so that the dill is pressed up against the side of the jar.

In a small saucepan, heat the vinegar, water, sugar, and salt until it starts to boil. Stir to dissolve salt and sugar.

Turn off the heat.

Carefully pour the brine over the vegetables, using a sterlilized funnel if desired. The level of the vinegar should come to the top of the jar and cover all the vegetables. Close the jar with the lid and wipe off the outside of the jar. Let stand on the kitchen counter until cooled to room temperature. Refrigerate for at least 24 hours. Can be stored in the refrigerator for up to 2 weeks, if they last that long.

Spicy Bahn Mi pickles

4 cloves garlic, peeled and crushed

2 radishes, washed and sliced

2 cucumbers, washed and cut into cubes

1 jalapeño pepper, washed and thinly sliced

2 carrots, peeled and sliced

Pickled cauliflower and carrot mix

4 cloves garlic, peeled and crushed

2 cups cauliflower florets

1 cup sliced carrot or carrot sticks

¼ large red onion, peeled and cut into slices or chunks

1 large sprig fresh dill

Pickled red onion and cucumber mix

4 cloves garlic, peeled and crushed

3 cups cucumber chunks or spears

1 cup red onion chunks

1 large sprig fresh dill

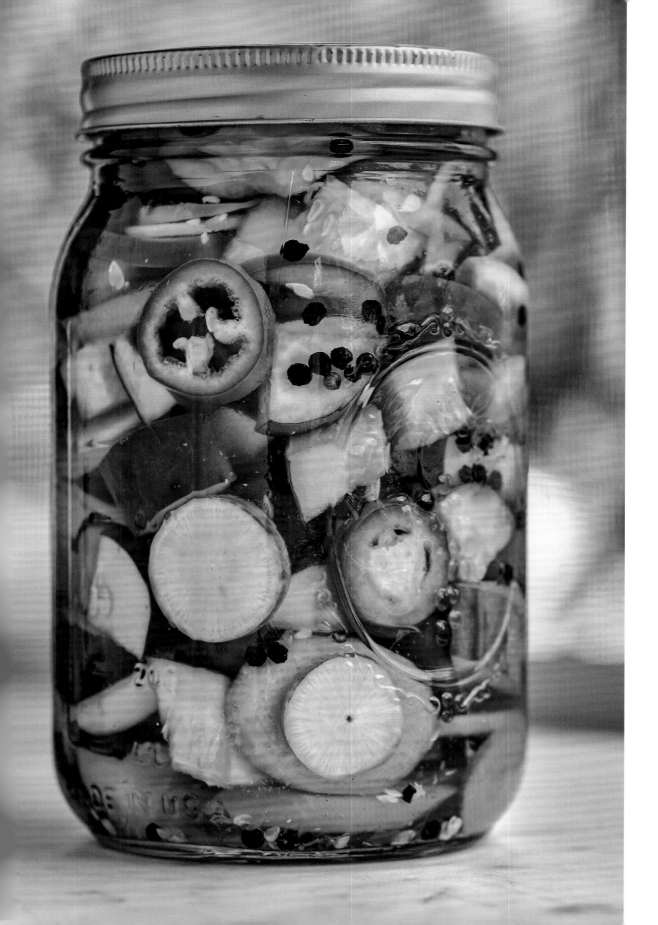

Buffalo Tofu

Serves 4 to 6

Shop for tofu in the refrigerated area of the natural or "organic" food department. You can serve this dish as an appetizer with sliced celery or as a suppertime entree with a slaw or salad. Buffalo sauce and hot sauce are not the same thing. You can buy Buffalo sauce already prepared, but why not make your own with your pantry of ingredients, since Buffalo sauce is almost always based on hot sauce, with the addition of some sort of liquid fat and other seasonings, such as garlic, vinegar, or cayenne pepper. For this recipe, pick your favorite sauce—either mild or spicy garlic.

Ingredients:

One 14-ounce package extra-firm tofu

2 tablespoons all-purpose flour

1 teaspoon garlic powder

½ teaspoon kosher salt

¼ teaspoon freshly ground black pepper

¼ cup canola oil

Celery sticks

Mild sauce

1 cup Frank's RedHot Sauce

¼ cup olive oil

1 tablespoon sugar

½ teaspoon garlic powder

¼ teaspoon cayenne pepper

¼ teaspoon kosher salt

Spicy garlic sauce

1 cup Frank's RedHot Sauce

¼ cup olive oil

1 tablespoon sugar

1 teaspoon garlic powder

½ teaspoon cayenne pepper

Directions:

First, press the excess moisture out of the tofu. Slice open the tofu package and drain off the water. Place the block of tofu on a plate and put the tofu box on top of the tofu. Fill the tofu box with items such as lemons or a can of beans or tomato sauce. This places gentle pressure on the tofu and presses out excess moisture. Let the tofu sit and press for about 15 minutes.

Meanwhile, whisk together the ingredients for the sauce of your choice and keep warm.

Remove the box from the top of the tofu and move the tofu to a cutting board. With a paper towel, pat the excess moisture off the surface of the tofu. Slice the tofu in half across the middle, like a bun. You now have two rectangular slices of tofu stacked on top of each other. Cut the tofu in half widthwise (down the middle). You now have 4 sections of tofu. Cut each section into 6 cubes.

In a shallow dish, mix the flour, garlic powder, salt, and pepper.

In a skillet, heat the canola oil over medium heat. Dredge cubes of tofu in the flour to coat. Cook the tofu cubes in batches, browning on the first side for about 5 minutes. With a spatula, turn the tofu and continue to cook for 3 to 4 minutes until the second side is brown and crispy. Move to a glass baking dish and keep warm in a 200°F oven. Just before serving, ladle warm buffalo sauce over the tofu cubes. Broil the tofu and sauce until hot and bubbly.

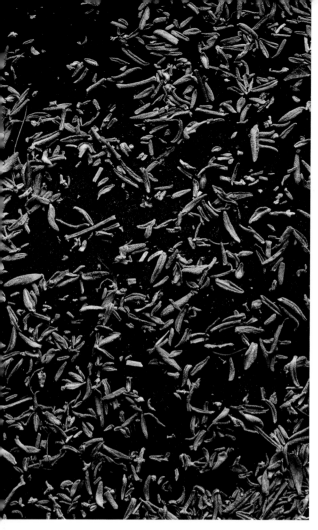

Olive Spread

Makes about 2 cups

This salty, versatile spread pairs well with roasted vegetables, grilled bread, fresh sliced bread, or fresh vegetables such as celery sticks, zucchini spears, or whole blanched green beans. It is also good as a spread on a wrap sandwich.

Ingredients:

¾ cup pitted Kalamata olives

¾ cup pitted green olives

¼ cup sliced almonds

1 clove garlic, sliced

¼ cup fresh parsley or basil

¼ teaspoon dried thyme

¼ cup olive oil

1 tablespoon water

Directions:

Place all ingredients in a food processor or blender. Mix until all ingredients are blended but still chunky. Serve at room temperature. Store in the refrigerator.

Frank's RedHot Sauce

According to their website, Frank's RedHot "original cayenne pepper sauce is made with a premium blend of aged cayenne peppers that add a kick of heat and a whole lot of flavor to your favorite foods." I chose Frank's for this book, and for the Buffalo Tofu recipe, because it's widely available and is the hot sauce used to create the original Buffalo wings created in Buffalo, New York, in 1964.

Green Hummus

Makes about 1 ½ cups

This simple, flavorful dip looks like guacamole. Serve with Skillet Croutons, page 79, pita chips, or sliced fresh vegetables. Save chickpea liquid to make a batch of Plant-Based Mayonnaise 1, page 48.

Ingredients:

One 15-ounce can chickpeas, drained,
   or 1 ½ cups cooked beans but reserve
   the cooking liquid

¼ cup olive oil

¼ cup tahini

2 tablespoons lemon juice
   (from about 1 lemon)

1 ½ teaspoons garlic powder

2 cups baby spinach or baby kale

¾ teaspoon kosher salt

⅛ teaspoon cayenne pepper

Directions:

Place all ingredients in a blender or food processor. Process until smooth. If needed, add up to ¼ cup of the chickpea liquid to adjust the consistency to desired thickness.

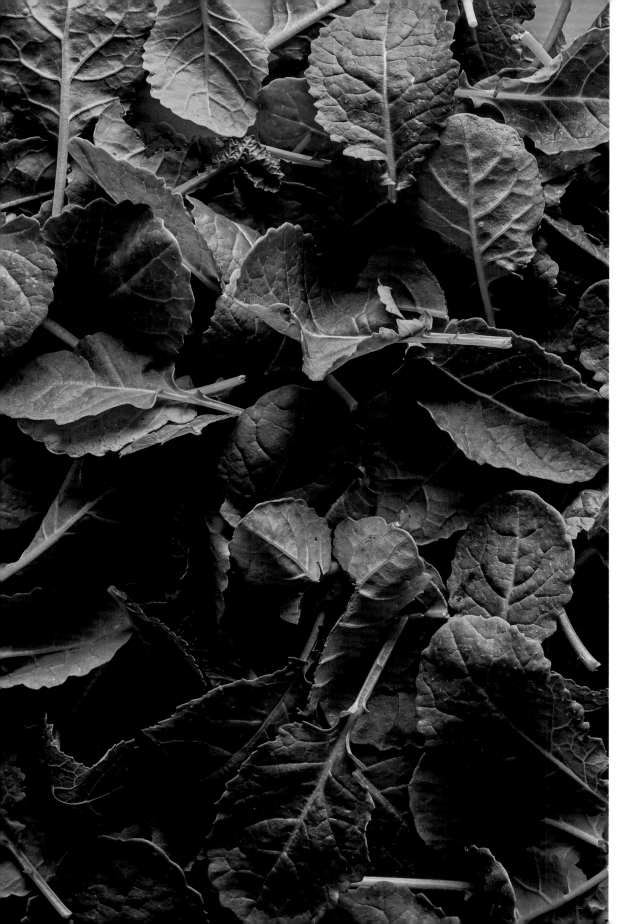

gluten free

Roasted White Bean Dip

Make about 2 cups

Roasted garlic and onion are more mellow than when uncooked and are sweeter too. Roasting the beans with the onions and garlic allows this dip to be served warm if desired.

Ingredients:

¼ cup olive oil, divided

½ small red onion, finely diced

2 cloves garlic, minced

One 15-ounce can great northern beans, or
1 ½ cups cooked great northern beans

¼ cup water

2 tablespoons lemon juice (from about 1 lemon)

¼ cup tahini

½ teaspoon kosher salt

Freshly ground black pepper

Directions:

Preheat oven to 375°F.

In an ovenproof saucepan or medium skillet, over medium heat, heat 2 tablespoons olive oil. Add the onion and cook for 5 minutes to soften the onion. Stir in the garlic, beans, and water. Place in oven and bake for 20 to 25 minutes or until starting to brown. Remove from oven and place beans in a blender or food processor. Add the lemon juice, tahini, remaining 2 tablespoons olive oil, and salt. Blend or process until smooth.

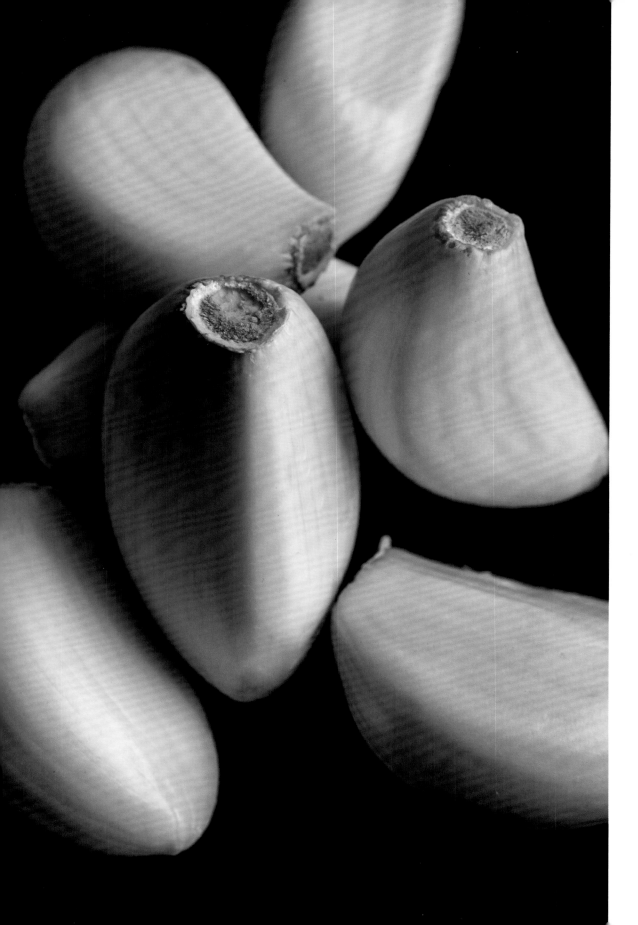

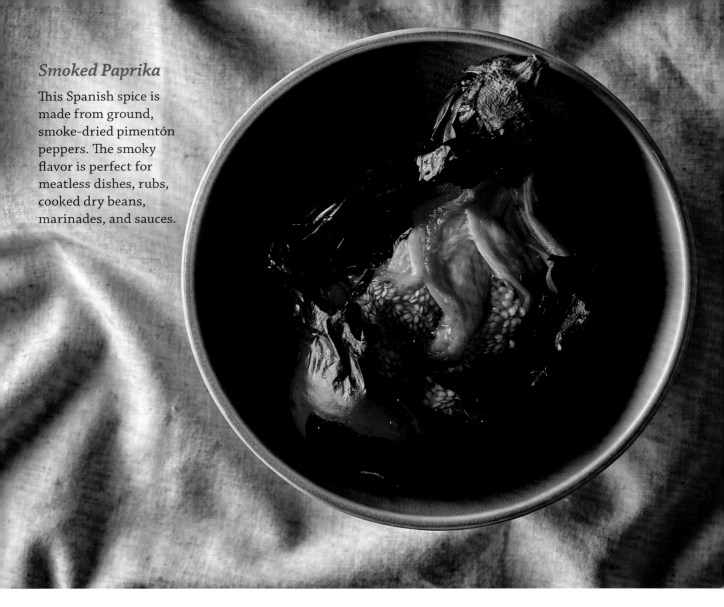

Smoked Paprika

This Spanish spice is made from ground, smoke-dried pimentón peppers. The smoky flavor is perfect for meatless dishes, rubs, cooked dry beans, marinades, and sauces.

gluten free

Smoky Eggplant Dip

Makes about 2 cups

Roast an eggplant over a gas flame or on a grill to "melt" or soften the interior of the eggplant and add a true smoky flavor. The smoked paprika adds an even smokier flavor. Alternatively, roast the eggplant in a hot oven. Serve with pita chips, whole-grain crackers, rice crackers, or thick sliced-vegetable.

Ingredients:

1 large globe eggplant, washed

¼ cup chopped roasted red pepper

¼ cup tahini

½ teaspoon garlic powder

2 tablespoons olive oil

2 tablespoons red wine vinegar

½ teaspoon smoked paprika

½ teaspoon kosher salt

¼ teaspoon red pepper flakes

Optional: chopped fresh parsley

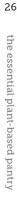

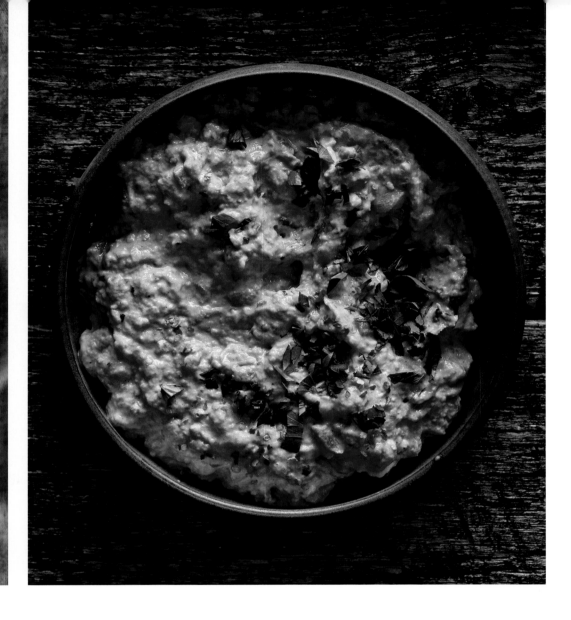

Directions:

Place a small baking rack over the gas flame of a stove or preheat a grill to medium-high. Wash and dry the eggplant. Place the eggplant over the gas flame. Use a pair of tongs to turn the eggplant periodically during cooking until the eggplant is soft on the inside and blackened on the outside. This takes about 20 to 25 minutes depending on the size of the eggplant.

Move the eggplant to a bowl and cover with foil. Set aside until cool enough to be handled without burning your fingers, about 15 minutes. The eggplant will continue cooking and will be even softer and mushier when the foil is removed.

Meanwhile, place the red pepper, tahini, garlic powder, olive oil, red wine vinegar, smoked paprika, salt, and red pepper flakes in a bowl and mix well.

Cut the eggplant open, scoop out the eggplant pulp, and put it into the bowl with the other ingredients. Mix well, stirring vigorously until the dip is smooth with chunks of red pepper and eggplant. The eggplant may remain just a little stringy, but the dip should be creamy in consistency. Serve warm or refrigerate and serve at a later time.

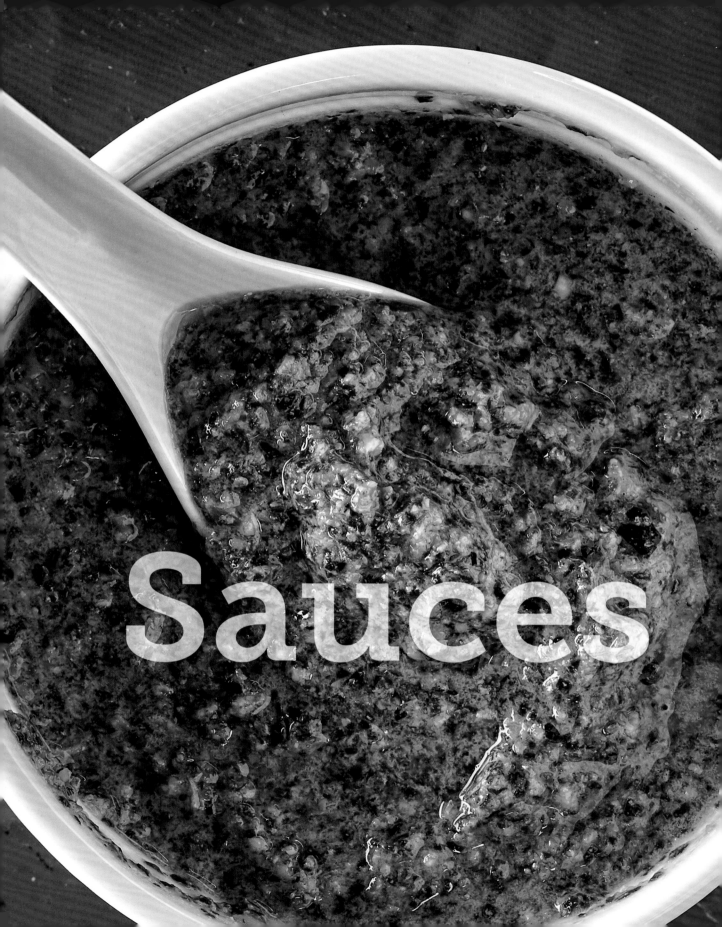

Sauces

Sauces often conjure up images of heavy, goopy liquids that cover up the real food underneath. This has changed for the modern cook. The approach with these "sauce" recipes is to provide a set of rubs, spice blends, and sauces that can be used in many different ways. With a pantry stocked with tomatoes, spices, nuts, herbs, vinegar, and olive oil, the combinations are almost limitless. To make the best use of this chapter, mix the rubs and spice blends ahead of time. Store them in an airtight container or jar, so they are ready when you need them. The tomato-based sauces on their own create a nice dish when served over Pan-Fried Tofu, page 157, any cooked whole grain, or pasta. And the Fresh Herb Vinaigrette, page 52, is fresh and flavorful. Making it ahead allows you to keep your grocery budget focused on pantry ingredients and not on buying jars and bottled of premade salad dressings and sauces.

❧ Recipes

Home-Blended Chili Powder and Curry Powder

Spicy Marinara Sauce

Tomato Curry Sauce

Fire-Roasted Tomato Salsa

Cashew Cream Sauce

Barbecue Sauce

Almond Curry Pesto

Kale Green Onion Pesto

Tahini Sauce

Plant-Based Mayonnaise, Two Ways

Enchilada Sauce

Fresh Herb Vinaigrette

Sriracha Peanut Sauce

Sweet Chile Vinaigrette

Ginger Sesame Vinaigrette

Home-Blended Chili Powder and Curry Powder

gluten free

With a pantry of spices, it's easy to make your own spice blends.

Chili powder

Makes 3 tablespoons

1 tablespoon smoked paprika

2 teaspoons cumin

2 teaspoons dried oregano

1 teaspoon garlic powder

1 teaspoon onion powder

½ teaspoon kosher salt

½ teaspoon cayenne pepper

Mix all ingredients and store in a small jar or another airtight container.

Curry powder

Makes 3 tablespoons

1 tablespoon coriander

1 tablespoon turmeric

1 teaspoon cumin

½ teaspoon freshly ground black pepper

¼ teaspoon powdered ginger

¼ teaspoon cayenne pepper

¼ teaspoon kosher salt

Mix all ingredients and store in a small jar or airtight container.

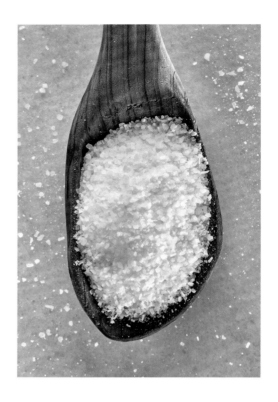

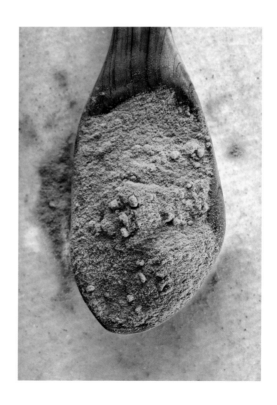

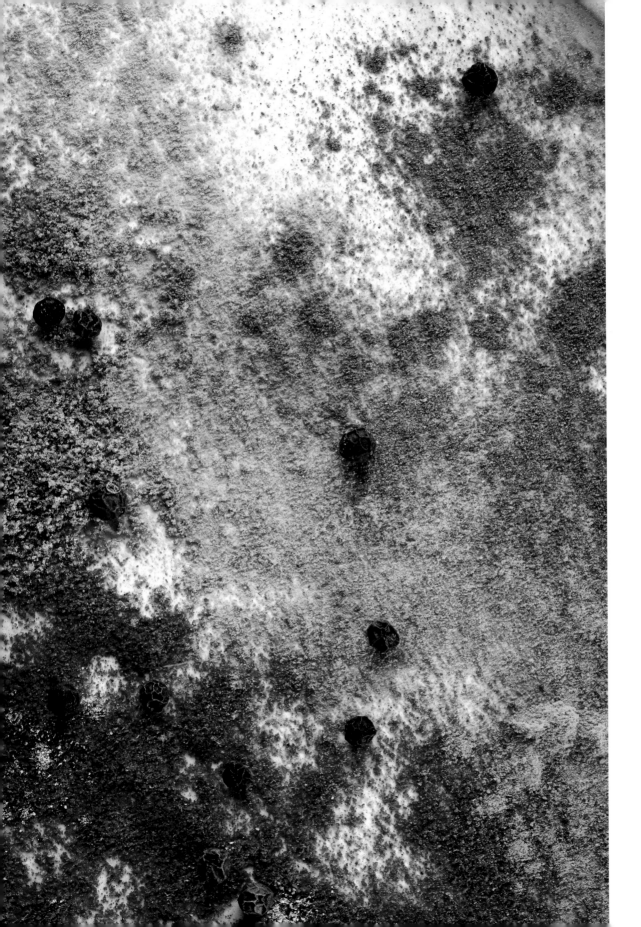

Spicy Marinara Sauce

Makes about 3 cups

This homemade version of marinara is quickly assembled from your pantry and replaces the need to buy a jar of marinara sauce.

Ingredients:

2 tablespoons olive oil

4 cloves garlic, finely chopped

¼ teaspoon red pepper flakes

¼ cup red wine

One 28-ounce can crushed tomatoes

2 tablespoons tomato paste

1 1/2 tablespoons dried basil

½ teaspoon dried thyme

1 tablespoon lemon juice (from about 1/2 lemon)

½ teaspoon kosher salt

¼ teaspoon freshly ground black pepper

Directions:

In a large skillet, heat the olive oil over medium-low heat. Add the chopped garlic and red pepper flakes and cook, stirring occasionally, for about 2 minutes. Do not allow the garlic to brown. Add the red wine and stir. Let simmer for about 1 minute to reduce the wine. Stir in the crushed tomatoes, tomato paste, basil, thyme, sugar, salt, and pepper. Bring to a simmer and cook, partially covered if it's blopping out of the pan too much, for about 30 minutes or until slightly thickened.

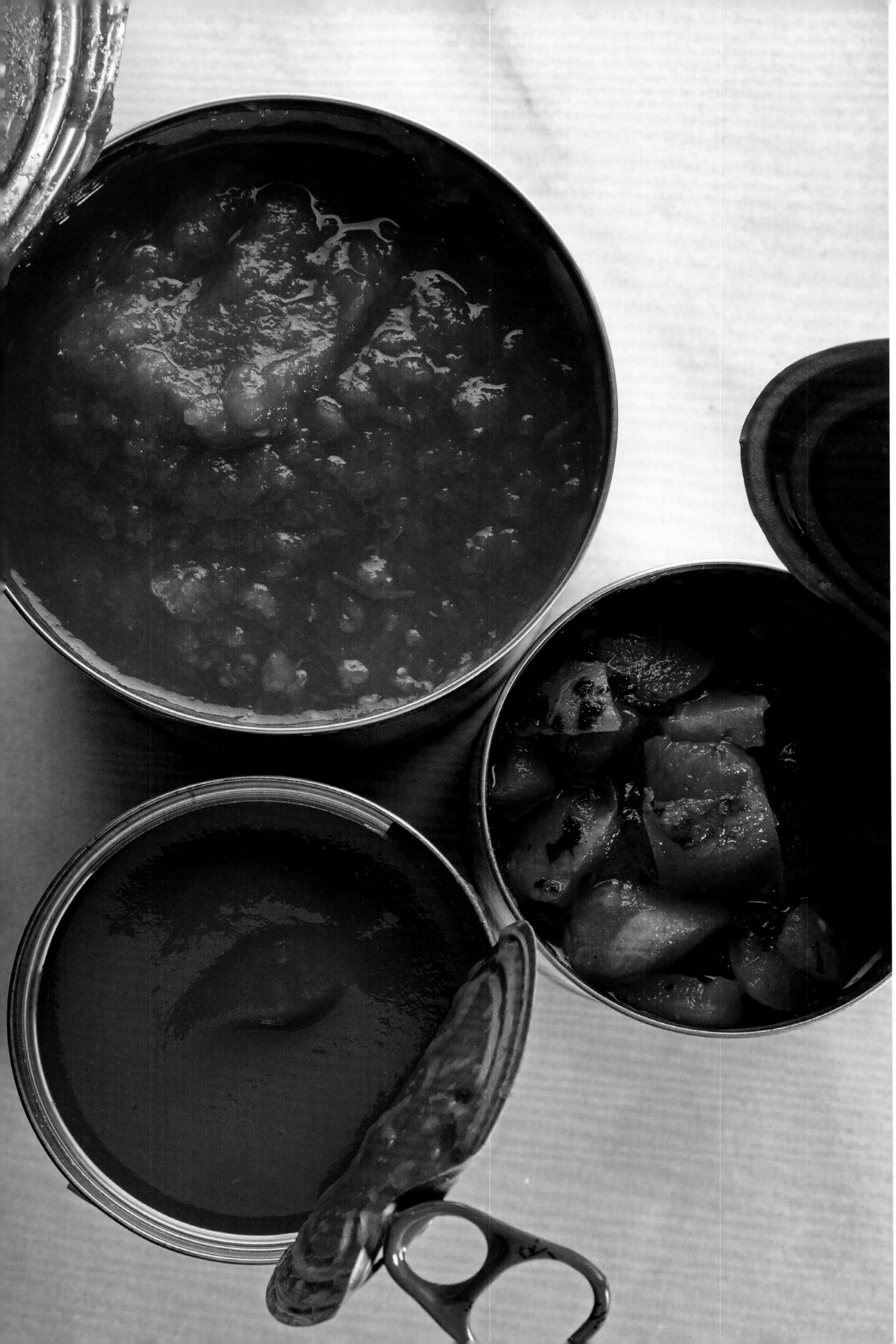

Tomato Curry Sauce

gluten free

Makes about 3 cups

This Indian-spiced tomato sauce is good with cooked chickpeas, Pan-Fried Tofu, page 157, or slices of cooked tempeh.

Ingredients:

2 tablespoons olive oil

1 tablespoon curry powder

½ teaspoon coriander

½ teaspoon cumin

½ teaspoon garlic powder

1 teaspoon kosher salt

½ teaspoon red pepper flakes

One 28-ounce can crushed tomatoes

1 tablespoon lemon juice (from about ½ lemon)

⅓ cup chopped fresh mint

Directions:

In a saucepan, heat olive oil over medium heat. Stir in the curry powder, coriander, cumin, garlic powder, salt, and red pepper flakes and mix well. Add the crushed tomatoes and lemon juice. Bring to a simmer and cook for about 30 minutes or until slightly thickened. Top with chopped fresh mint before serving.

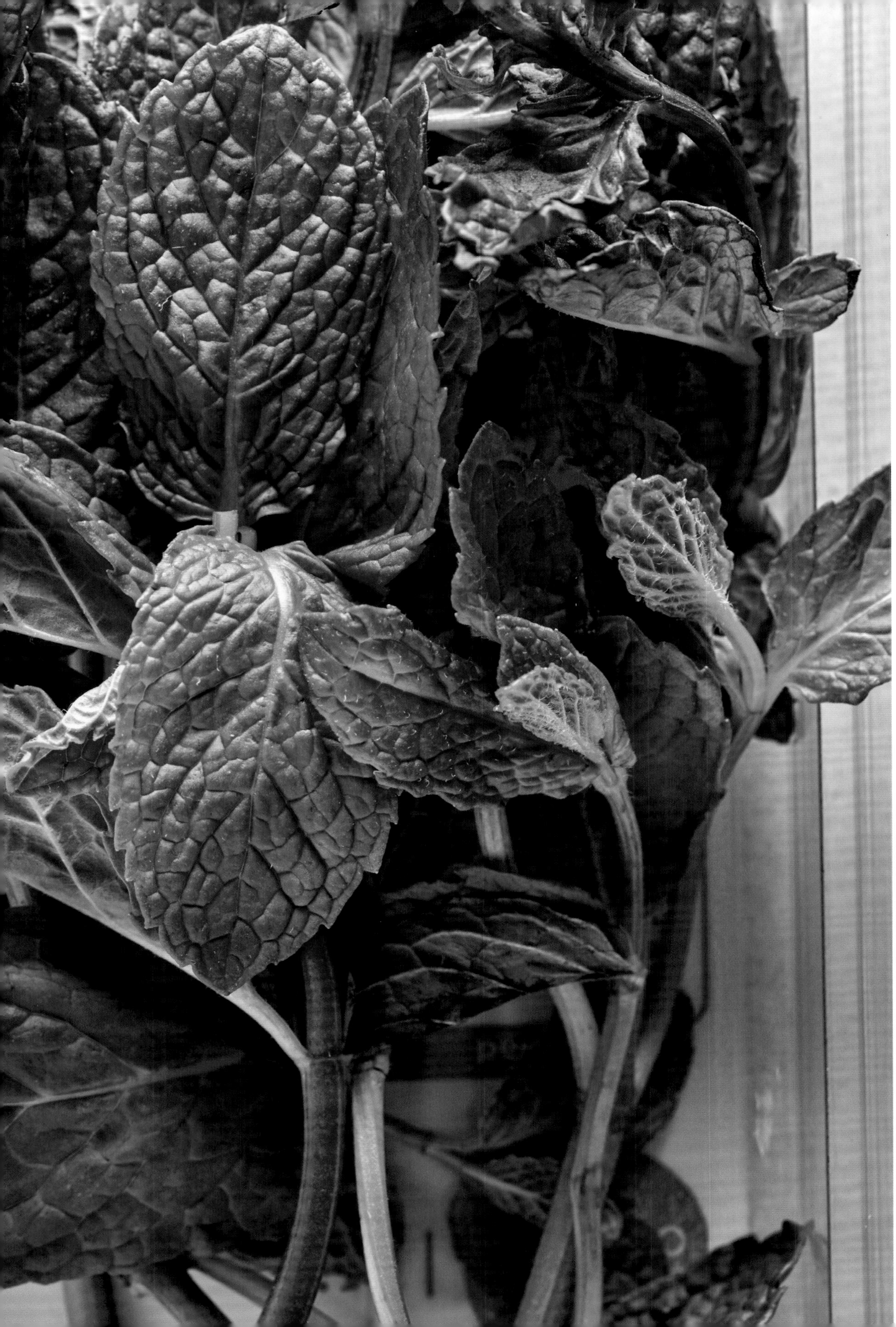

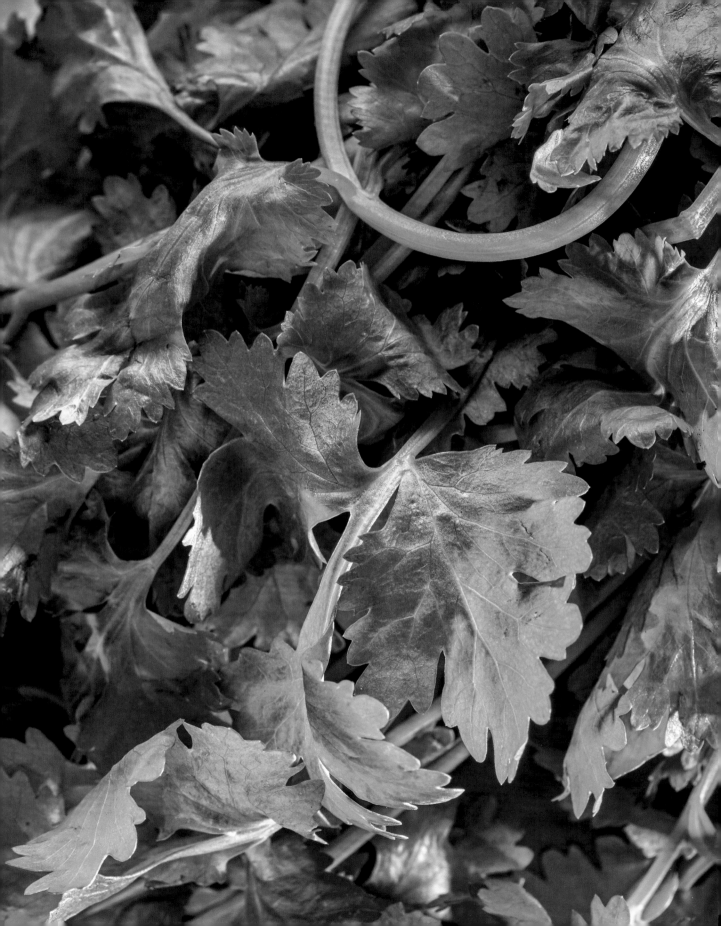

gluten free

Fire-Roasted Tomato Salsa

Makes about 1 ½ cups

Made with canned tomatoes and canned green chiles, this salsa pairs well with Smoky Red Beans and Rice, page 144, or Kidney Bean Burgers, page 148. For the best flavor, refrigerate for at least one hour before serving. If using red onion, soak it in a bowl of water for thirty minutes to kill the sharp onion flavor, if desired.

Ingredients:

One 14 ½-ounce can fire-roasted diced tomatoes

One 4-ounce can chopped green chiles

¼ cup finely chopped red or green onion

2 cloves garlic, minced

¼ cup chopped fresh cilantro

1 tablespoon olive oil

Juice of 1 lime

½ teaspoon kosher salt

Optional: 1 ½ teaspoon hot sauce

Directions:

Mix all ingredients together in a bowl, for a chunky salsa. For a smooth salsa, blend in a food processor. Store in refrigerator.

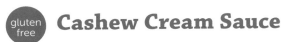

Cashew Cream Sauce

Makes 2 cups

For a smooth sauce, it's essential to soak the cashews. If you plan to make this for supper, soak the cashews in the morning when you make your coffee. This sauce can be used on pasta, in soups, for scalloped potatoes, or as a cream sauce in vegetable lasagna.

Ingredients:

1 cup raw cashews

1 ½ cups water, plus more for soaking cashews

2 tablespoons olive oil

4 cloves garlic, minced or ½ teaspoon garlic powder

Zest of 1 lemon

1 tablespoon lemon juice (from about ½ lemon)

¾ teaspoon kosher salt

¼ teaspoon freshly ground black pepper

Directions:

Place raw cashews in a glass or other heat-proof bowl. Cover with hot water. Cover the bowl and soak overnight or at least 8 hours. This softens the cashews to make them easy to blend.

To make the cashew cream, drain the cashew soaking water. Using a blender, mix the cashews and 1 ½ cups water on high speed for 1 minute. Scrape down the sides and process again until smooth and creamy. Add the olive oil, garlic, lemon zest, lemon juice, salt, and pepper. Blend well. Store refrigerated for up to 3 days.

Raw Cashews

Raw cashews aren't roasted or salted. At my supermarket, raw cashews are sold with bulk foods, although in other markets they may be sold in the produce department or the natural foods section of the store. It is possible to substitute unsalted roasted cashews if you can't find raw. You can use either whole cashews or pieces, although the pieces may be more economical.

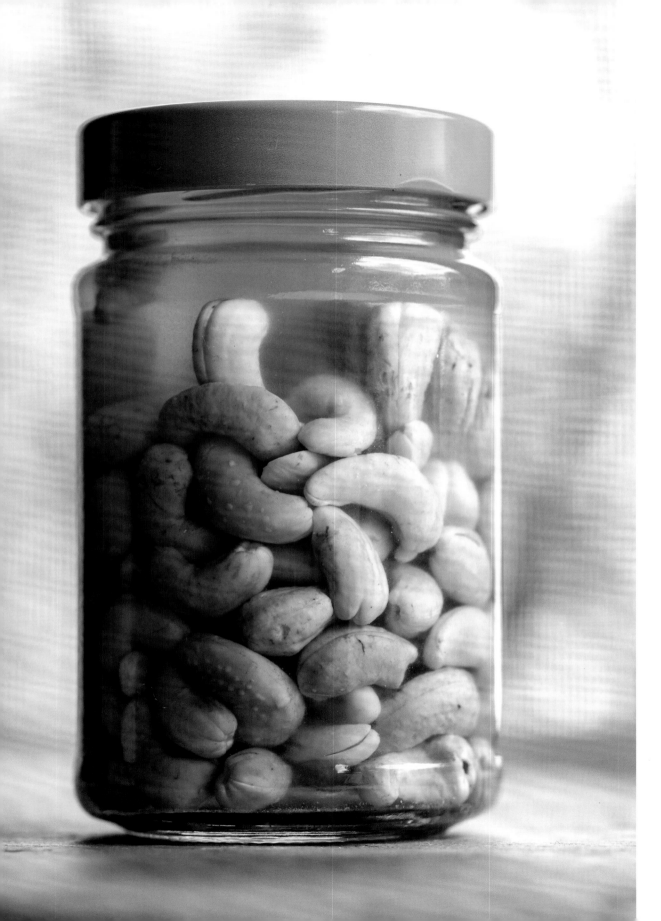

39

Barbecue Sauce (gluten free)

Makes 1 cup

This multiuse, tomato-based sauce stores well in the refrigerator. In the world of barbecue, Memphis utilizes a tomato-based sauce, and this is similar. Mix in chopped chipotle in adobo for added heat and smoke flavor. Used as a base in Barbecue Lentils, page 126, this sauce is also good with any cooked white bean; Pan-Fried Tofu, page 157; or slices of cooked tempeh.

Ingredients:

3 tablespoons olive oil

3 tablespoons brown sugar

1 tablespoon honey

1 tablespoon apple cider vinegar

2 teaspoons chili powder

1 teaspoon smoked paprika

1 teaspoon kosher salt

½ teaspoon garlic powder

½ teaspoon onion powder

⅛ teaspoon cayenne pepper

One 8-ounce can tomato sauce (1 cup)

Optional: 1 tablespoon chopped chipotle in adobo

Directions:

In a small saucepan, heat the olive oil over medium-low heat. Add the brown sugar, honey, vinegar, chili powder, smoked paprika, salt, garlic powder, onion powder, and cayenne pepper. Stir to make a paste. Whisk in the tomato sauce and bring to a gentle boil. Simmer for about 15 minutes. Serve warm or let cool and refrigerate in a bottle, jar, or other airtight container.

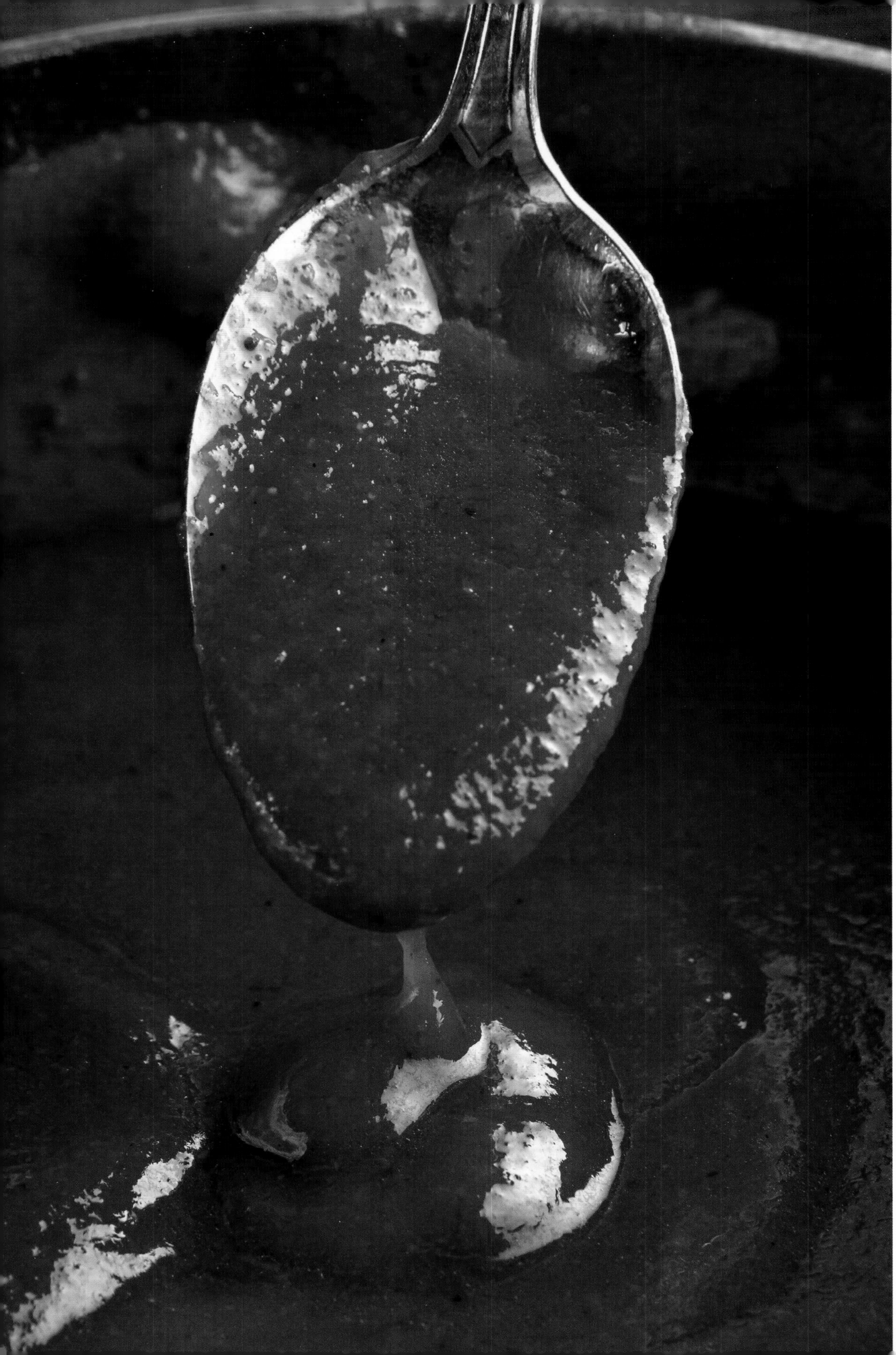

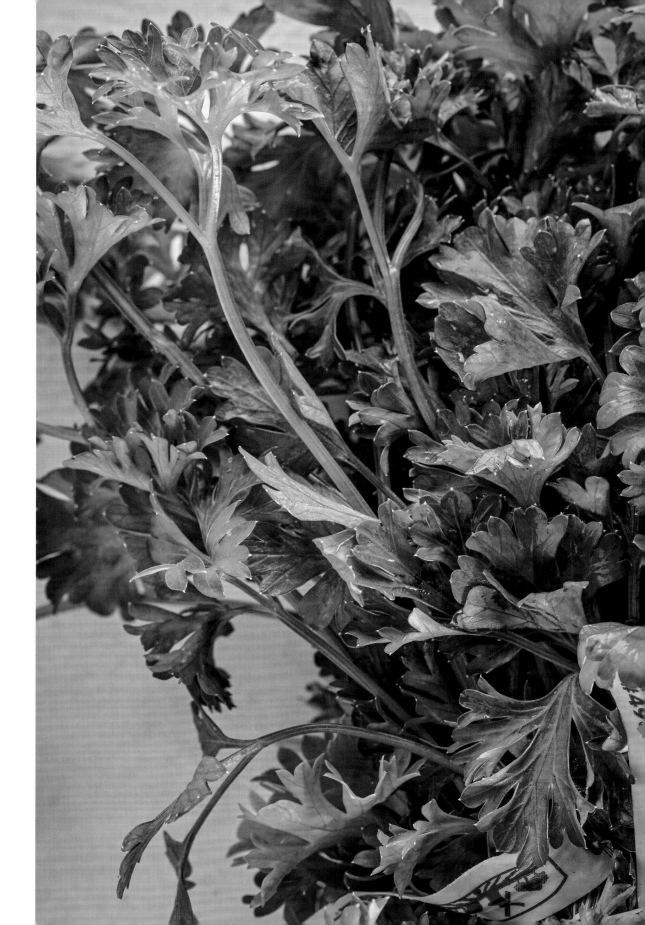

Almond Curry Pesto

 gluten free

Makes about 1 cup

Sweet, salty, nutty, and herby, this pesto can be used on hot pasta or gluten-free pasta, cooked chickpeas, rice, or cauliflower.

Ingredients:

½ cup sliced almonds

¼ cup dried cranberries or golden raisins

½ cup fresh cilantro, roughly chopped

¼ cup fresh parsley, roughly chopped

¼ cup olive oil

2 tablespoons red wine vinegar

1 ½ teaspoons curry powder

¼ teaspoon kosher salt

Directions:

Place all ingredients in a blender or food processor. Pulse until well blended but still chunky.

Storing Pesto

Use the pesto immediately or spoon it into a container to store. By pouring a thin layer of olive oil on the top of the pesto, you can keep the herbs from turning dark.

Curry Powder

This spice blend is readily available in most supermarkets. The blend commonly contains spices such as ground turmeric (which creates the yellow color), cumin, coriander, and black pepper. In India, blends of spices are customized by home cooks and blended at home for use in curries. These blends are sometimes called Garam Masala or Madras Curry Powder. You can also blend your own Curry Powder, page 30, from spices in your pantry.

Kale Green Onion Pesto

Makes about 2 cups

There are multiple uses for pesto, including stirred into mayonnaise for a dip or thinned out with extra olive oil and lemon juice to use as a vinaigrette for salad. This recipe is also used on the Roasted Japanese Sweet Potato dish, page 122, or it can be tossed with hot cooked pasta or gluten-free pasta.

Ingredients:

2 cups baby kale

¼ cup fresh basil leaves

2 thin green onions, white part, and
   2 inches of the green part, thinly sliced

1 clove garlic, peeled and crushed

1 tablespoon lemon juice (from about ½ lemon)

½ cup chopped walnuts

½ cup olive oil

1 teaspoon kosher salt

Directions:

Place all ingredients in a food processor or blender. Pulse until well blended. Use as desired.

   To store, place the pesto in a storage container. Pour a thin layer of olive oil over the pesto. Cover and refrigerate. The thin layer of oil keeps the pesto bright green by blocking exposure to air.

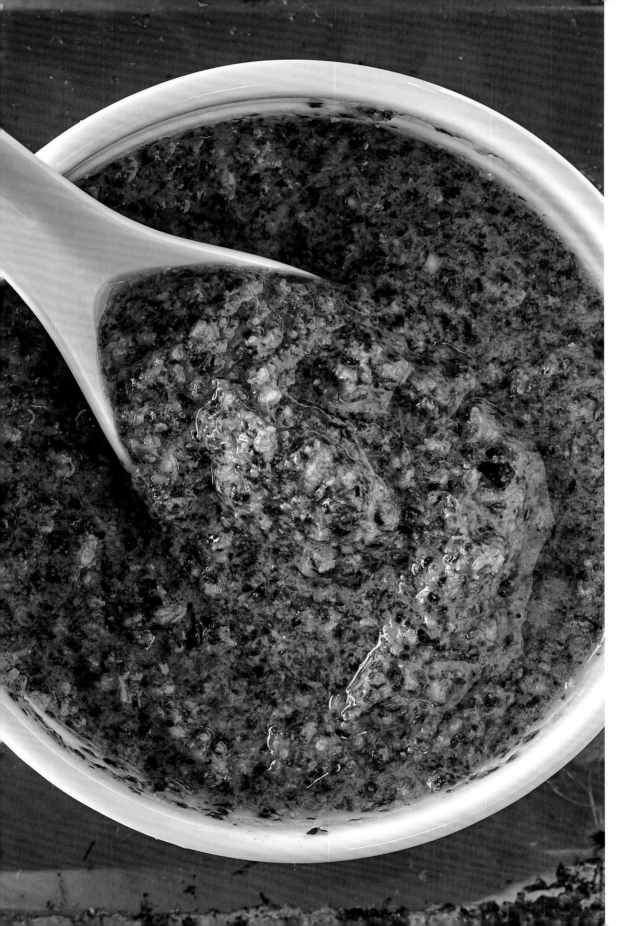

45

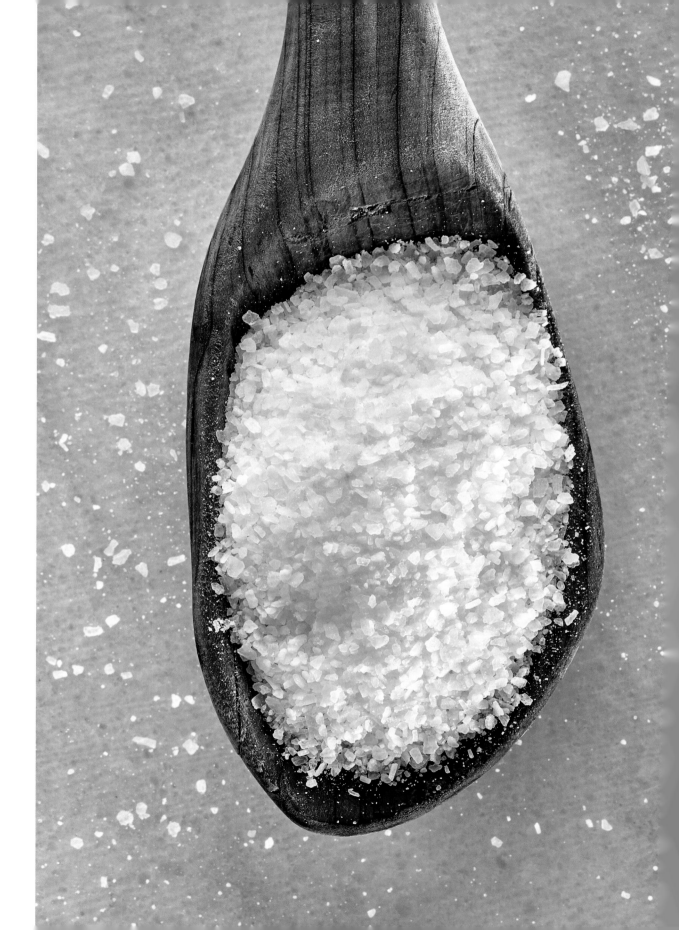

Tahini Sauce

gluten free

Makes about ½ cup

This sauce pairs well with Kidney Bean Burgers, page 148, and is used as a dressing on Apple and Celery Salad, page 96. It would also be nice tossed with fresh spring greens or sliced, seeded cucumbers.

Ingredients:

¼ cup lemon juice

3 tablespoons tahini

2 tablespoons olive oil

2 tablespoons water

1 garlic clove, minced

¼ teaspoon kosher salt

Optional: pinch cayenne pepper

Directions:

Whisk all ingredients together in a small bowl. Store in the refrigerator.

Tahini

Like peanut butter is to peanuts, tahini is to sesame seeds— a creamy, off-white paste made from sesame seeds. Stir in the oil if it separates.

gluten free

Plant-Based Mayonnaise, Two Ways

These two creamy sauces can be used in place of mayonnaise and are both made from plant-based ingredients.

Plant-Based Mayonnaise 1

Makes 1 cup

Aquafaba, or the liquid from cooking legumes, is the replacement for egg in this mayonnaise. *Aqua* is Latin for water and *faba* is Latin for bean. In this recipe, I use chickpea liquid, which has a thick consistency. The theory is that the starch and protein in the liquid acts as an egg, and these particles bind with the oil to make mayonnaise. The secret to success with this recipe is to drip drop the oil in at first very, very, slowly to allow the aquafaba and oil to emulsify. If you add the oil too fast, the liquid turns white but doesn't thicken. The oil can be streamed in a little quicker toward the end, once the emulsion is formed. You won't believe how much this tastes and looks like mayonnaise.

Ingredients:

¼ cup aquafaba (liquid from canned chickpeas)

1 teaspoon lemon juice (from about ½ lemon)

½ teaspoon Dijon mustard

½ teaspoon kosher salt

¾ cup neutral vegetable oil such as canola

Directions:

In a blender, mix the aquafaba, lemon juice, mustard, and salt. With the blender running, very slowly drip drop the first ¼ cup of oil into the running blender. It should start to look thick, and the sound of the whirring will even change as the mixture thickens. Then add the remaining ½ cup oil very slowly in a thin stream and process until all the oil is added and the mixture is creamy and thick.

Plant-Based Mayonnaise 2

Makes 1 cup

This savory sauce is based on silken tofu. These ingredients do not form a creamy emulsion, like plant-based mayonnaise 1, so it's a little easier to make.

Ingredients:

8 ounces silken tofu

2 tablespoons olive oil

1 tablespoon lemon juice (from about ½ lemon)

1 teaspoon Dijon mustard

¼ teaspoon kosher salt

Freshly ground black pepper

Directions:

Blend all ingredients in a food processor or blender.

Other variations include the following.

Sriracha mayonnaise

To every 1 cup mayonnaise add:

2 tablespoons sriracha

Vegan caesar dressing

To every 1 cup mayonnaise add:

1 clove garlic, minced

2 tablespoons lemon juice (from about 1 lemon)

2 tablespoons capers

Garlic mayonnaise or aioli

To every 1 cup mayonnaise add:

2 clove garlic, minced

Cayenne garlic mayonnaise

To every 1 cup mayonnaise add:

2 clove garlic, minced

⅛ teaspoon cayenne pepper

Green goddess mayonnaise

To every 1 cup mayonnaise add:

1 clove garlic, sliced

¼ cup chopped green onion

½ cup minced flat-leaf Italian parsley

½ cup minced fresh basil leaves

¼ teaspoon kosher salt

Cilantro lime jalapeño mayonnaise

Use lime juice instead of lemon juice in the recipe and once blended, add:

2 cloves garlic minced

¼ cup fresh minced cilantro

2 tablespoons chopped jalapeño, include seeds for more heat

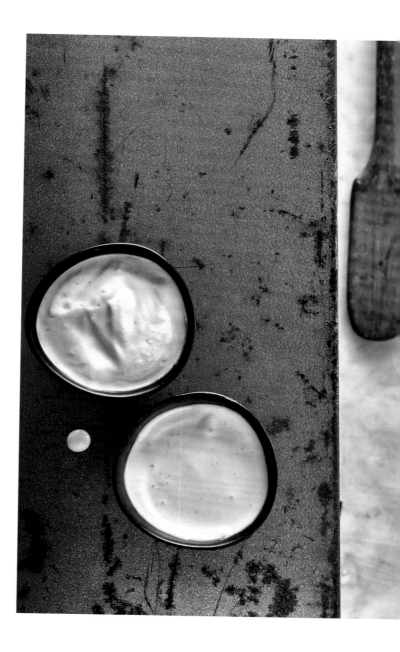

Silken Tofu versus Traditional Tofu

Tofu comes in two main types: silken and regular. Silken tofu is softer in consistency than standard tofu, and it reminds me of tofu jello. Silken tofu may be packaged in a shelf-stable box that doesn't require refrigeration. When shopping for silken tofu, check the refrigerated or grocery section of the natural food department. Use blended or pureed silken tofu in dishes that require a thick and creamy texture.

sauces

Enchilada Sauce

Make about 3 cups

A spicy, tomato-based sauce, this recipe is good served with Pan-Fried Tofu, page 157, and rice. Add chopped chipotle in adobo for smoke and heat, but vary the amount depending on how spicy you want the final sauce.

Ingredients:

2 tablespoons olive oil

½ to 1 tablespoon chopped chipotle in adobo

2 tablespoons chili powder

1 tablespoon cumin

1 teaspoon smoked paprika

1 teaspoon garlic powder

½ teaspoon kosher salt

One 28-ounce can tomato sauce

Directions:

In a saucepan over low heat mix the olive oil, chipotle in adobo, chili powder, cumin, smoked paprika, and garlic powder. Stir in the tomato sauce and bring to a low boil. Reduce heat and keep warm until needed.

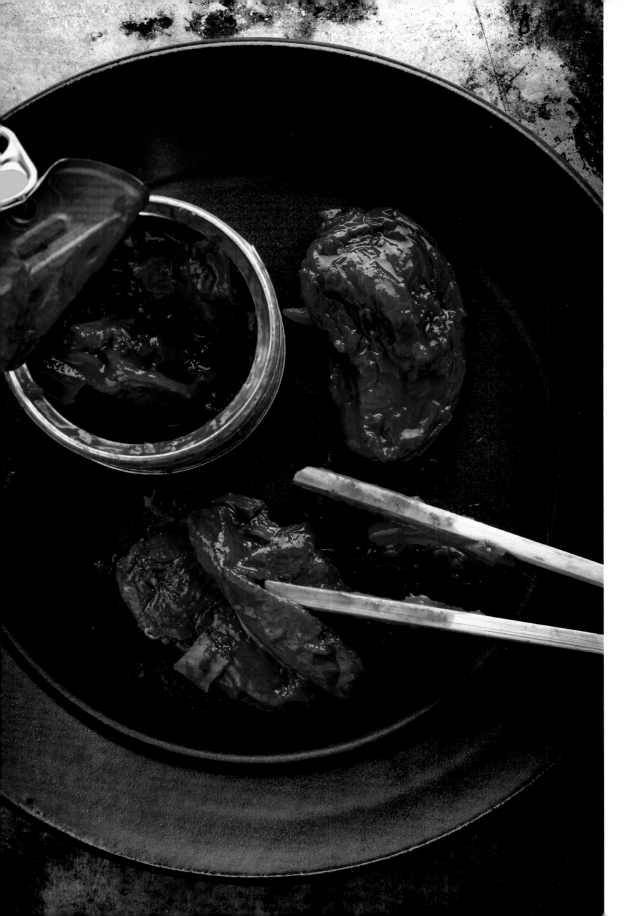

Fresh Herb Vinaigrette

Makes about 1 cup

If you want to create a house vinaigrette good for chopped vegetables and leafy green salads, this just might be it.

Ingredients:

1 cup parsley

½ cup fresh basil leaves or 1 teaspoon
    dried basil

½ teaspoon dried oregano

2 cloves garlic, peeled

¼ cup red wine vinegar

¾ cup olive oil

¾ teaspoon kosher salt

¼ teaspoon pepper

Directions:

Place all ingredients in a blender. Pulse to chop the herbs. Blend well to make a bright green vinaigrette.

Vinaigrette

A vinaigrette is a classic mixture of oil and vinegar and seasonings such as mustard, herbs, and spices. It can be used to dress salads and as a marinade. Some like to call a vinaigrette a salad dressing, which it is, but a vinaigrette can be used for more than just salads.

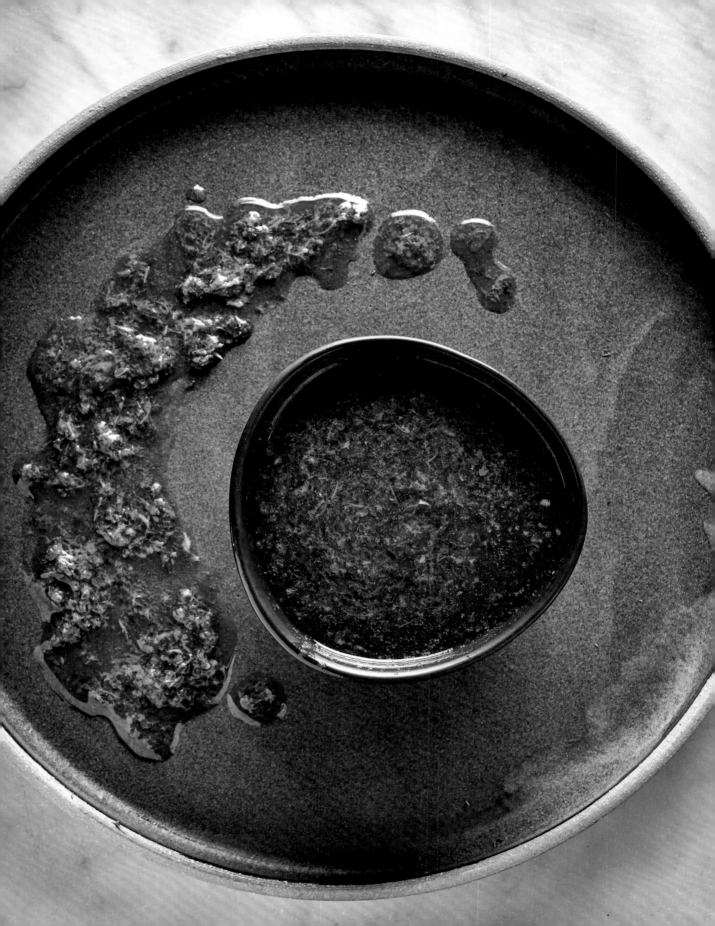

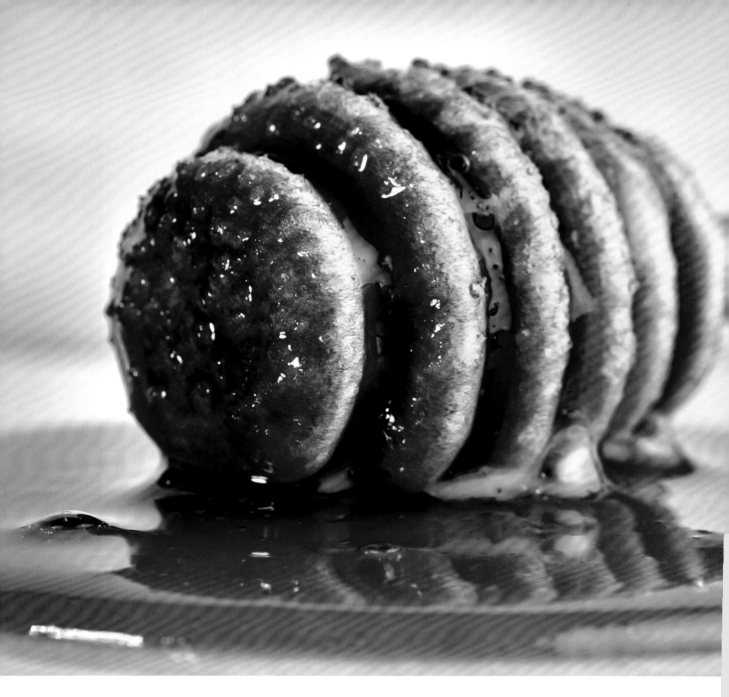

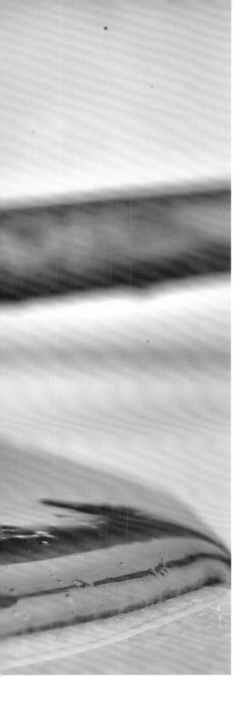

Sriracha Peanut Sauce

Makes about 1 cup

A nice dressing for noodle or cabbage salads, this sauce is very versatile. It's also good served with assorted sautéed vegetables such as carrot, green beans, zucchini or summer squash, broccoli, red cabbage, or brussels sprouts on a bed of rice or mixed with thin spaghetti and topped with slices of red pepper, cucumber, and fresh chopped mint for a refreshing salad.

Ingredients:

¼ cup peanut butter

2 cloves garlic, peeled and minced

3 tablespoons canola oil

2 tablespoons honey

2 tablespoons apple cider vinegar

2 tablespoons lime juice (from about 1–2 limes)

2 tablespoons water

1 tablespoon fresh grated ginger root
    or ginger paste

1 tablespoon reduced-sodium soy sauce
    or tamari

1 tablespoon sriracha

1 teaspoon kosher salt

Directions:

In a bowl, whisk together the ingredients. Store in the refrigerator.

Sweet Chile Vinaigrette

Makes about ⅔ cup

Ingredients:

¼ cup water

2 tablespoons apple cider vinegar

2 tablespoons honey

1 tablespoon olive oil

2 tablespoons lime juice (from about 1–2 limes)

1 tablespoon fresh grated ginger root
  or ginger paste

2 cloves garlic, minced

½ teaspoon red pepper flakes

1 teaspoon sriracha

Directions:

In a small bowl, combine the water, vinegar, and honey. Whisk just to combine and dissolve the honey. Whisk in the oil, lime juice, ginger, garlic, red pepper flakes, and sriracha, and combine until well blended.

Sriracha

Made from chile peppers, vinegar, garlic, sugar, and salt, sriracha is a hot sauce named after a city on the coast of Thailand, named *Si Racha*. Keep a bottle in the refrigerator to use in recipes or as a spicy ketchup to add flavor and heat to roasted vegetables, eggs, or noodle bowls.

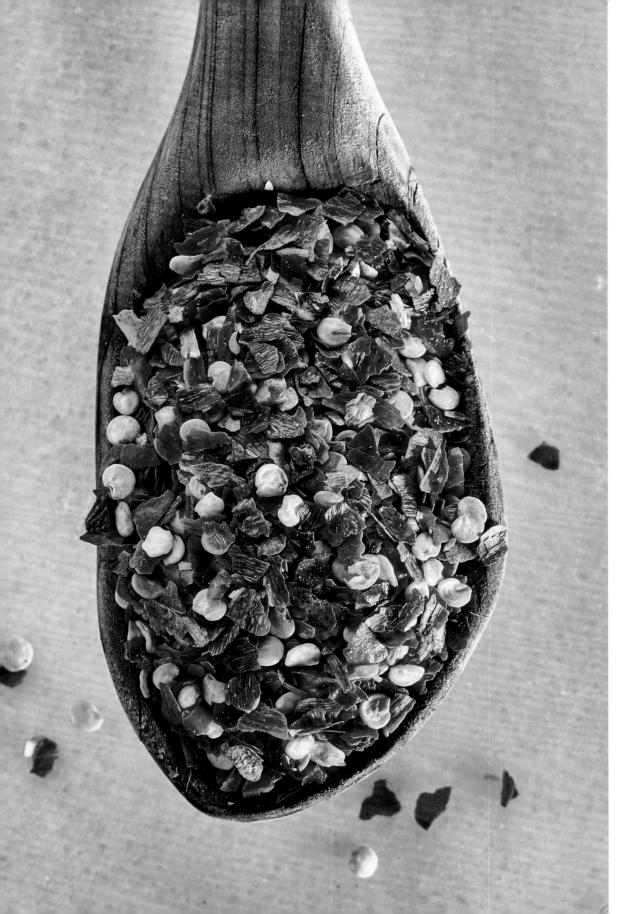

Ginger Sesame Vinaigrette

Makes about ⅓ cup

Ingredients:

2 tablespoons canola oil

1 tablespoon toasted sesame oil

1 tablespoon apple cider vinegar

1 tablespoon honey

1 tablespoon fresh grated ginger root
   or ginger paste

2 cloves garlic, peeled and minced

1 teaspoon reduced-sodium soy sauce
   or tamari

¼ teaspoon freshly ground black pepper

Directions:

In a small bowl, whisk the ingredients
together until smooth.

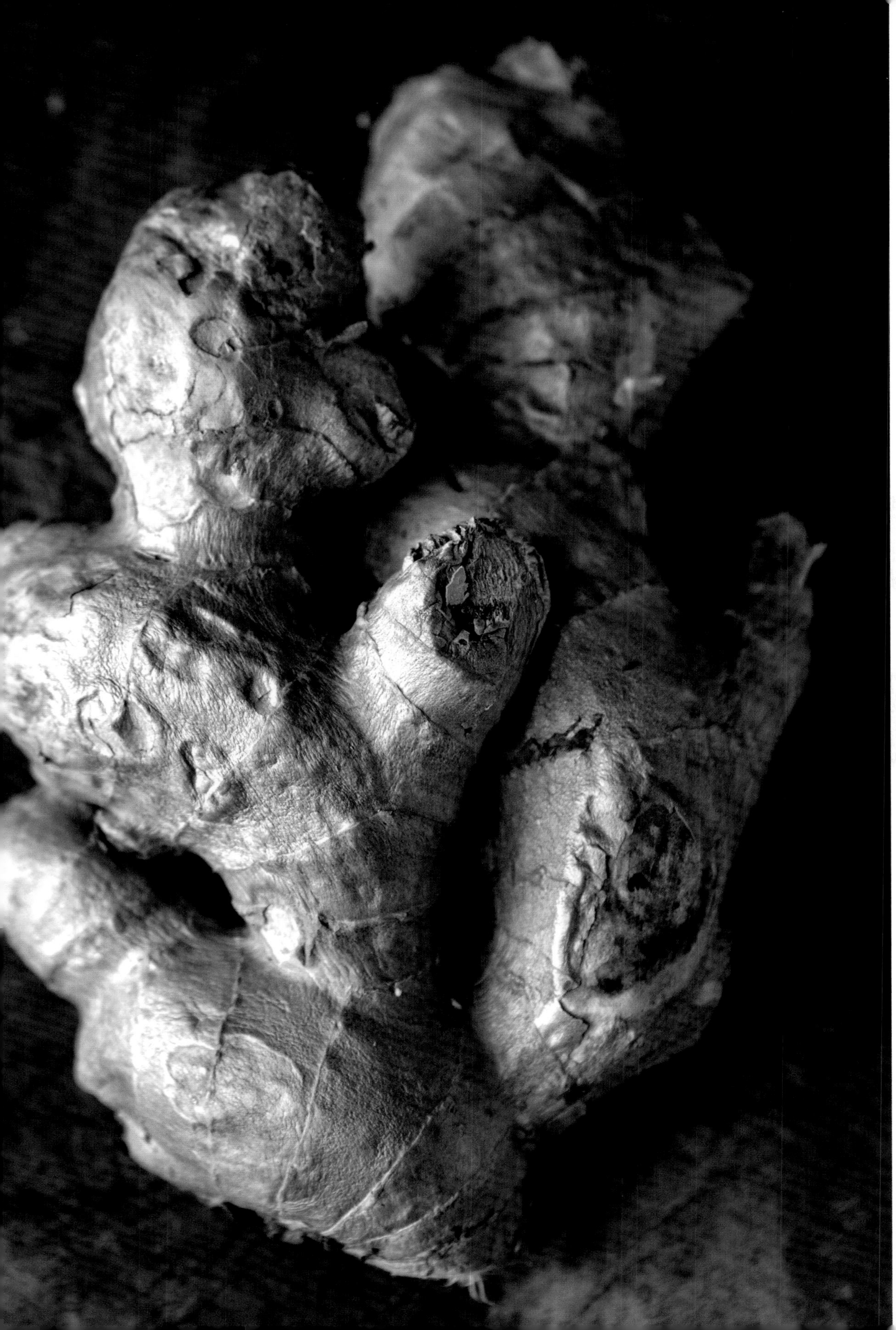

Soups

Soup is the ultimate home-cooked meal. And a hearty soup with chunky ingredients can be filling enough for the main course of a meal, while a pureed soup may need a sandwich or salad on the side. Any soup filled with beans, grains, and vegetables simmers unattended and allows the cook to do other things while the soup cooks. And the aroma! This communicates to anyone in and around the kitchen that suppertime is going to be good. For plant-based cream soups, cashew cream provides the richness, and the soup base allows for improvisation with other vegetables.

❧ Recipes

Curried Red Lentil, Quinoa, and Apple Soup

Vegetable Kale Soup

Lentil Barley Soup

Ginger Coconut Carrot Soup

Tomato, White Bean, and Spinach Soup

Cashew Cream of Broccoli Soup

Tortilla Soup

Curried Red Lentil, Quinoa, and Apple Soup

Makes 8 cups

Red lentils cook quickly but turn a yellow color when cooked. The apples and quinoa add a nice body to the soup. Rice can be substituted for the quinoa, but if brown rice is used, increase the cooking time to forty-five minutes.

Ingredients:

2 tablespoons olive oil

½ medium onion, finely chopped

1 medium apple, cored and
    cut into small pieces

2 tablespoons honey

1 ½ tablespoons curry powder

½ teaspoon coriander

1 teaspoon kosher salt

¼ teaspoon cayenne pepper

1 cup red lentils

¼ cup quinoa, rinsed

One 13 ½ ounce can regular or
    lite coconut milk

4 cups water

Optional: chopped fresh cilantro

Directions:

In a saucepan, heat the olive oil. Add the onion and apple and cook until tender and starting to brown, about 8 minutes. Stir in the honey, curry powder, coriander, salt, and cayenne pepper. Mix well to blend. Add the red lentils, quinoa, coconut milk, and water. Bring to boil, reduce to simmer, and cook for 30 minutes until the lentils are soft. Serve topped with optional fresh cilantro.

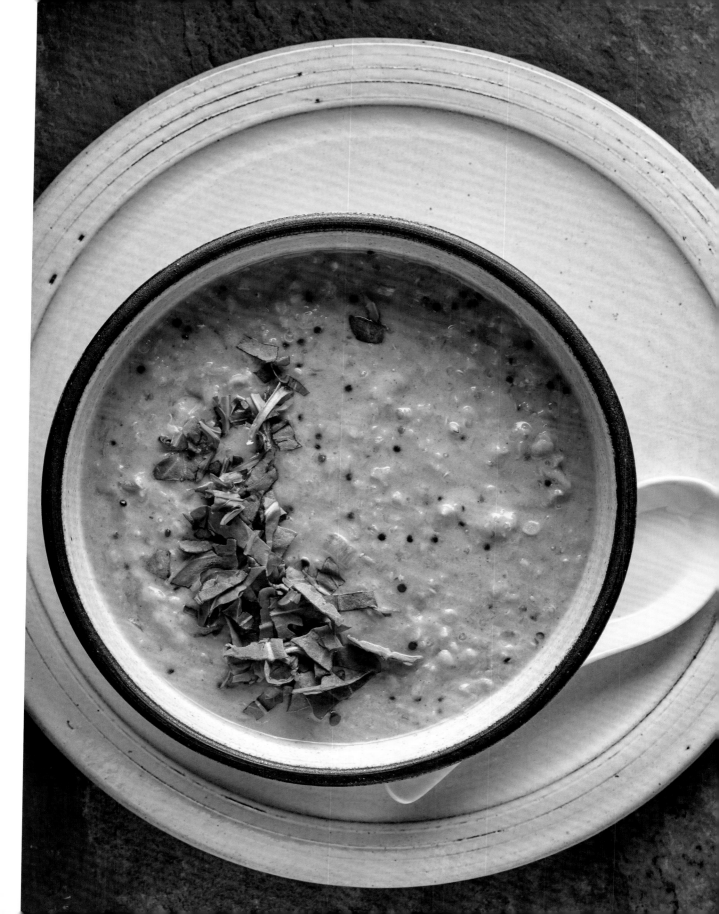

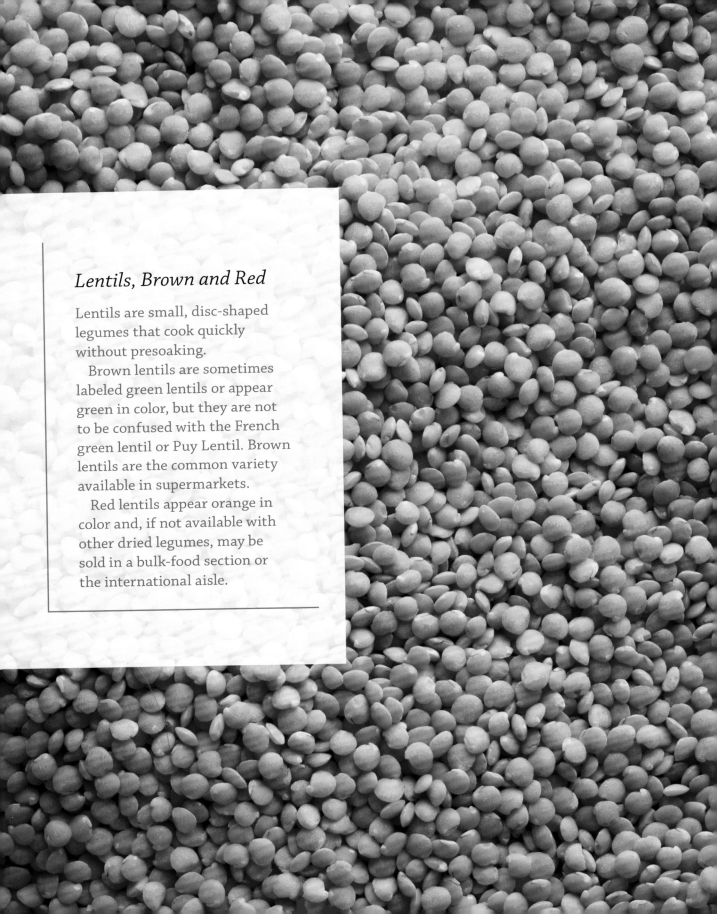

Lentils, Brown and Red

Lentils are small, disc-shaped legumes that cook quickly without presoaking.

Brown lentils are sometimes labeled green lentils or appear green in color, but they are not to be confused with the French green lentil or Puy Lentil. Brown lentils are the common variety available in supermarkets.

Red lentils appear orange in color and, if not available with other dried legumes, may be sold in a bulk-food section or the international aisle.

Vegetable Kale Soup

gluten free

Makes about 8 cups

Chock full of spices and vegetables, this soup is my go-to way to enhance store-bought broth for a warming vegetable soup.

Ingredients:

2 tablespoons olive oil

1 medium onion, chopped (about 1 cup)

3 ribs celery, thinly sliced

2 cups chopped kale

2 red or yellow potatoes, diced (about 2 cups)

4 cloves garlic, minced

2 teaspoons smoked paprika

1 teaspoon ground turmeric

1 teaspoon dried thyme

½ teaspoon kosher salt

½ teaspoon freshly ground black pepper

One 15-ounce can kidney or red beans, drained, or 1 ½ cups cooked beans

6 cups vegetable broth

Directions:

In a Dutch oven heat the olive oil over medium heat. Add onion and celery and cook, stirring occasionally until softened, about 5 minutes. Stir in the kale, potato, garlic, paprika, turmeric, thyme, salt, and pepper. Stir and cook for about 1 minute to blend ingredients and to soften the garlic. Stir in the beans and broth. Bring to a gentle boil, reduce heat, and simmer, partially covered, for about 30 minutes. Season to taste with salt and pepper before serving.

Lentil Barley Soup (gluten free)

Makes about 6 cups

This simple, lentil soup achieves a lot of its flavor from the garlic and smoked paprika. Substitute brown rice for barley if desired.

Ingredients:

1 tablespoon olive oil

4 cloves garlic, peeled and minced

2 teaspoons smoked paprika

1 ½ teaspoons dried thyme

¼ teaspoon cayenne pepper

1 cup brown lentils

¼ cup pearl barley

4 cups reduced-sodium vegetable broth

3 cups water

2 tablespoons tomato paste

¼ teaspoon kosher salt

¼ teaspoon freshly ground pepper

Directions:

In a soup pan, heat the olive oil over medium heat. Stir in the garlic and smoked paprika. Let the garlic cook briefly until fragrant. Stir in the thyme, cayenne pepper, lentils, and barley and coat with the oil and spices. Add the broth, water, and tomato paste. Stir to combine well. Bring to a boil, reduce heat, and simmer uncovered, for 55 to 65 minutes or until the lentils and barley are soft. Season with salt and pepper. Serve hot with a drizzle of olive oil.

Tomato Paste

Recipes often call for small quantities of tomato paste. When you open a can, chances are you'll have a lot left over. Here are a few solutions: If available, buy tomato paste in a squeeze tube that looks like a tube of toothpaste. In my supermarket it's sold in the International Aisle near the Italian food. With a tube, you can dispense small quantities, put cap back on the tube, and store the tube in the refrigerator. It's there when you need it. Alternatively, open one small can of tomato paste. Use what you need and spoon the remaining tomato paste in one-tablespoon quantities on a cookie sheet. Freeze them and then store in a zip-top bag in the freezer.

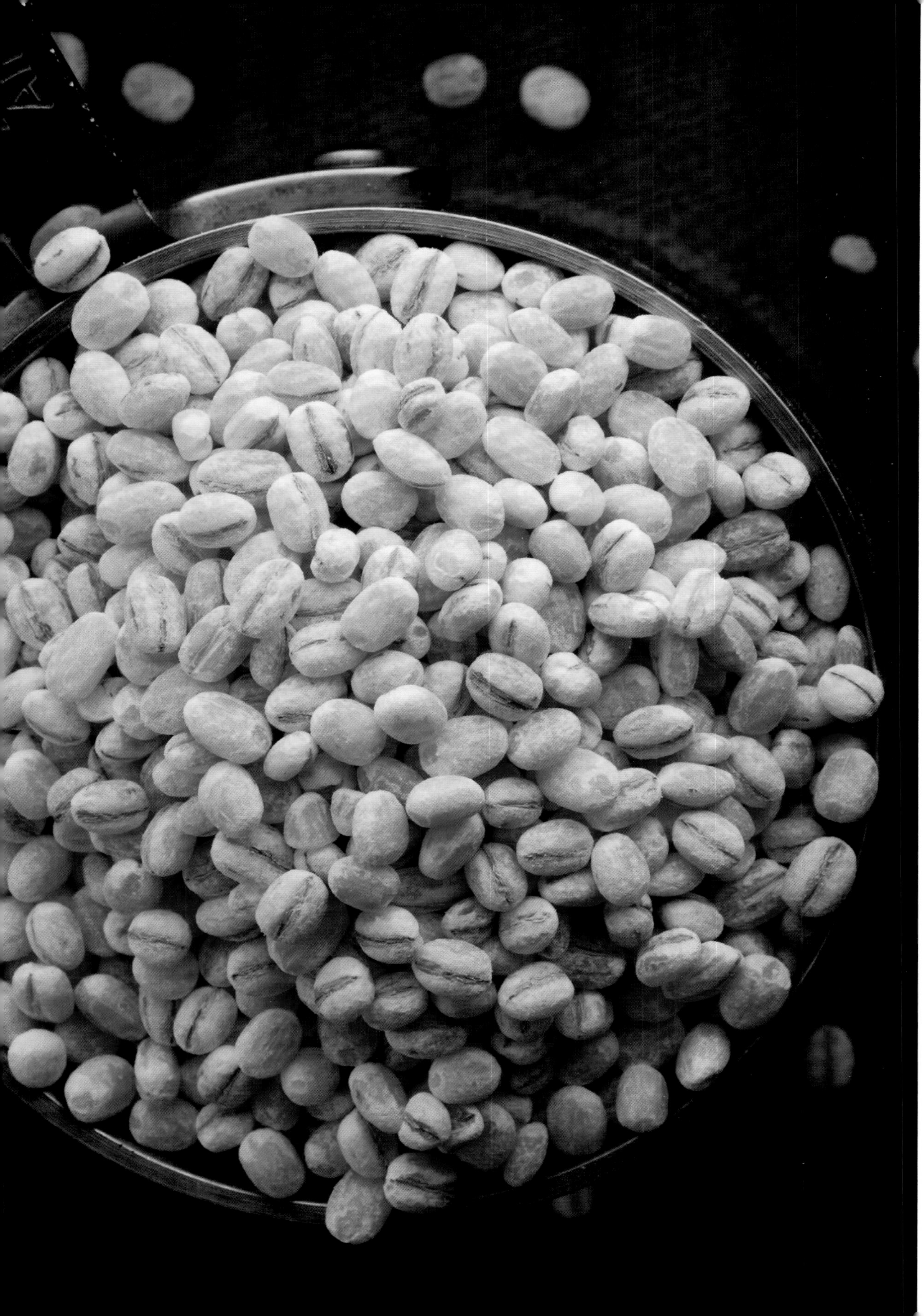

Ginger Coconut Carrot Soup

gluten free

Makes about 6 cups

This smooth, pureed carrot soup makes a meal when paired with Tofu Eggless Salad sandwiches, page 83; Sweet and Spicy Curried Chickpea Salad, page 80; or Barbecue Lentil "sloppy joes," page 126.

Ingredients:

2 tablespoons olive oil

1 medium onion, diced

4 cloves garlic, finely chopped

8 carrots, peeled and sliced
  (about 4 cups carrot slices)

1 tablespoon fresh grated ginger root or ginger
  paste or 1 ½ teaspoons powdered ginger

1 teaspoon kosher salt

⅛ teaspoon cayenne pepper

1 tablespoon honey

3 cups vegetable broth

One 13 ½ ounce can regular or lite coconut milk

Directions:

In a saucepan heat olive oil over medium heat. Add the onion and cook for about 5 minutes until lightly browned. Stir in the garlic and carrots. Cook, stirring occasionally, for 5 more minutes until the carrots start to soften and turn brown. Add the ginger, salt, and cayenne pepper. Stir well to coat the carrots in the spices. Add the honey, vegetable broth, and coconut milk. Bring to a simmer and cook for 20 minutes until carrots are soft.

With caution due to the heat of the soup, use a blender or immersion blender to puree the soup until smooth. Serve hot. Garnish with thinly sliced green onion tops and a drizzle of honey if desired.

Fresh Ginger Paste

Fresh ginger paste is sold in tubes or small bottles in the produce section of large supermarkets. It's perfect for cooks who enjoy the flavor of fresh ginger but want to skip the step of grating or chopping fresh ginger. Store the tube or bottle in the refrigerator.

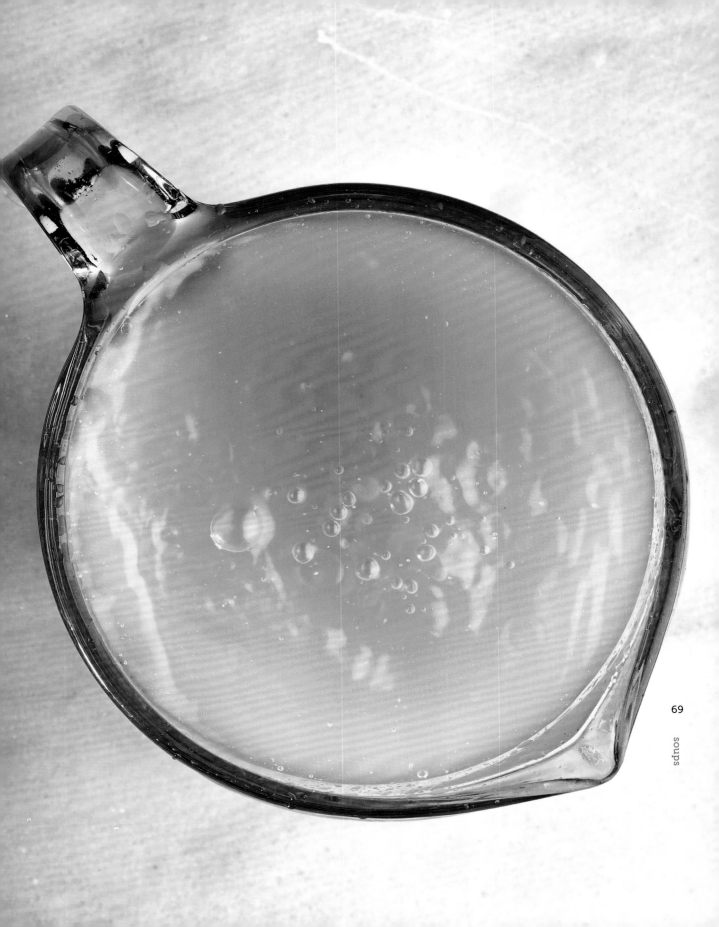

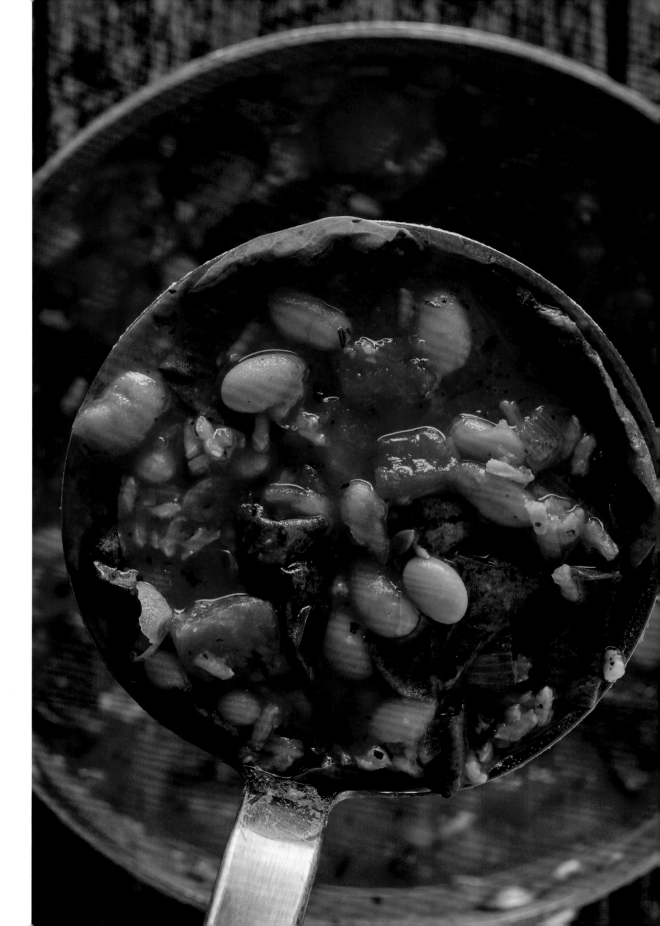

the essential plant-based pantry

Tomato, White Bean, and Spinach Soup

gluten free

Makes about 6 cups

For added richness and flavor, drizzle with olive oil or top with Kale Green Onion Pesto, page 44, before serving.

Ingredients:

2 tablespoons olive oil

1 medium onion, peeled and finely diced (about 1 cup)

4 cloves garlic, minced

½ teaspoon dried thyme

½ teaspoon dried basil

3 cups vegetable broth

One 15-ounce can fire-roasted diced tomatoes with their juice

One 15-ounce can great northern beans, drained and rinsed, or 1 ½ cups cooked beans

½ cup brown rice or pearled barley

¾ teaspoon kosher salt

½ teaspoon freshly ground black pepper

4 cups baby spinach leaves

Directions:

In a soup pan, heat the olive oil over medium heat. Stir in the onion and let cook for about 8 minutes until softened and starting to brown. Add garlic, thyme, and basil and stir well until the garlic is fragrant. Stir in the broth, tomatoes, beans, rice, salt, and pepper. Stir to combine well. Bring to a boil, reduce heat to simmer, and cook, uncovered, for 45 minutes, stirring occasionally. Add the baby spinach and cook for 10 more minutes. Season with salt and pepper.

Cashew Cream of Broccoli Soup

gluten free

Makes about 6 cups

Soaked raw cashews are used to create a cashew cream. This is used as the base for this soup, providing a rich and plant-based "cream." Raw cashews can be found in a bulk food area, the produce department, or the natural food section of the supermarket. Alternatively, substitute 1 ¼ cups unsweetened, plain cashew milk for the cashew cream.

To make a different variety of cream of vegetable soup, you can vary the vegetable. Substitute 2 cups chopped tomatoes, sliced mushrooms, frozen green peas, or sliced celery for the broccoli to make cream of tomato, mushroom, pea, or celery soup.

Ingredients:

1 cup raw cashews

1 ½ cups water, plus more for soaking

2 tablespoons olive oil

½ medium onion, peeled and diced

2 cups chopped broccoli florets
   (from about 1 pound)

¼ teaspoon garlic powder

¾ teaspoon dried thyme

1 teaspoon kosher salt

¾ teaspoon freshly ground black pepper

4 cups vegetable broth

Directions:

Place raw cashews in a glass or other heat-proof bowl. Cover with 1 inch hot water. Cover the bowl and soak overnight or at least 8 hours. This softens the cashews to make them easy to blend.

In a large sauce-pan heat olive oil. Add the onion and cook over medium heat until browned and translucent, about 6 to 8 minutes. Add the broccoli, garlic powder, thyme, salt, and pepper, and stir just to combine. Add broth and bring to a boil. Reduce the heat to a simmer, and cook uncovered for 10 minutes until the broccoli is cooked but crisp-tender and still a nice bright green color.

To make the cashew cream, drain the cashew soaking water. Using a blender, mix the cashews and 1 ½ cups of water on high speed for 2 minute. Scrape down the sides and continue to process until smooth and creamy.

When the broccoli is cooked, stir the cashew cream into the broccoli soup. Simmer for 5 minutes. Season with salt and pepper and serve hot.

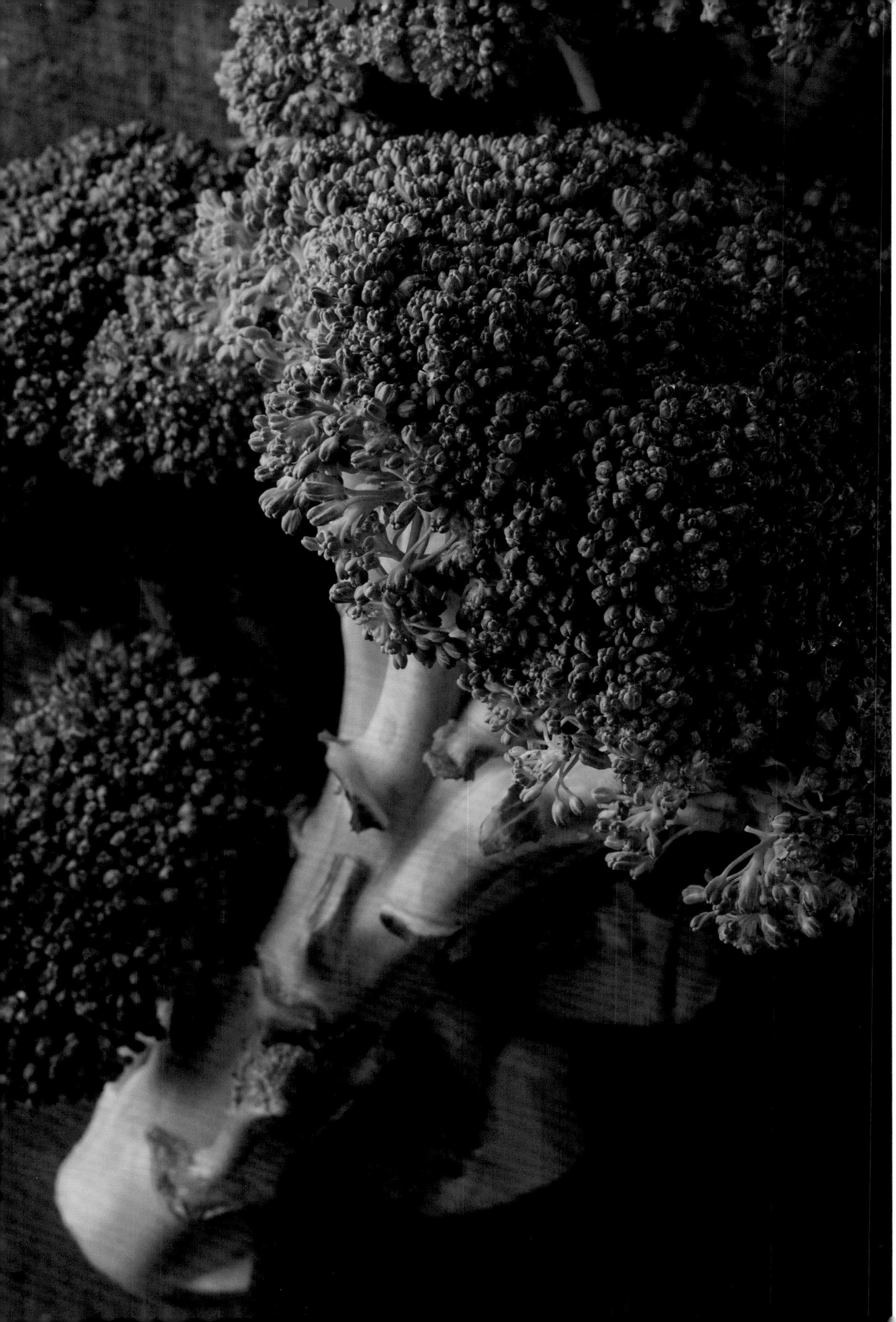

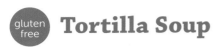

Tortilla Soup

Serves 6 to 8

This soup is good but, of course, is even better with crushed corn tortilla chips, sliced jalapeño, diced avocado, lime wedges, and fresh chopped cilantro.

Ingredients:

2 tablespoons olive oil

1 medium onion, peeled and diced (about 1 cup)

4 cloves garlic, minced

1 tablespoon chopped chipotle in adobo

½ cup red lentils

1 teaspoon chili powder

1 teaspoon smoked paprika

1 teaspoon cumin

½ teaspoon coriander

½ teaspoon kosher salt

Two 15-ounce cans black beans, drained, or 3 cups cooked beans

One 15-ounce can fire-roasted diced tomatoes with their juice

4 cups vegetable broth

Salt and freshly ground black pepper to taste

Optional: crushed corn tortilla chips, sliced jalapeno, diced avocado, lime wedges, chopped fresh cilantro

Directions:

In a saucepan heat olive oil over medium heat. Add the onion and cook for about 5 minutes until lightly browned. Stir in the garlic and chipotle in adobo. Cook for 1 minute until garlic is fragrant. Add the lentils, chili powder, smoked paprika, cumin, coriander, salt, black beans, fire-roasted tomatoes, and broth. Stir well and bring to a gentle boil. Reduce heat and simmer, uncovered, for about 25 to 30 minutes until the lentils are soft. Season to taste with salt and pepper and serve with assorted toppings on the side.

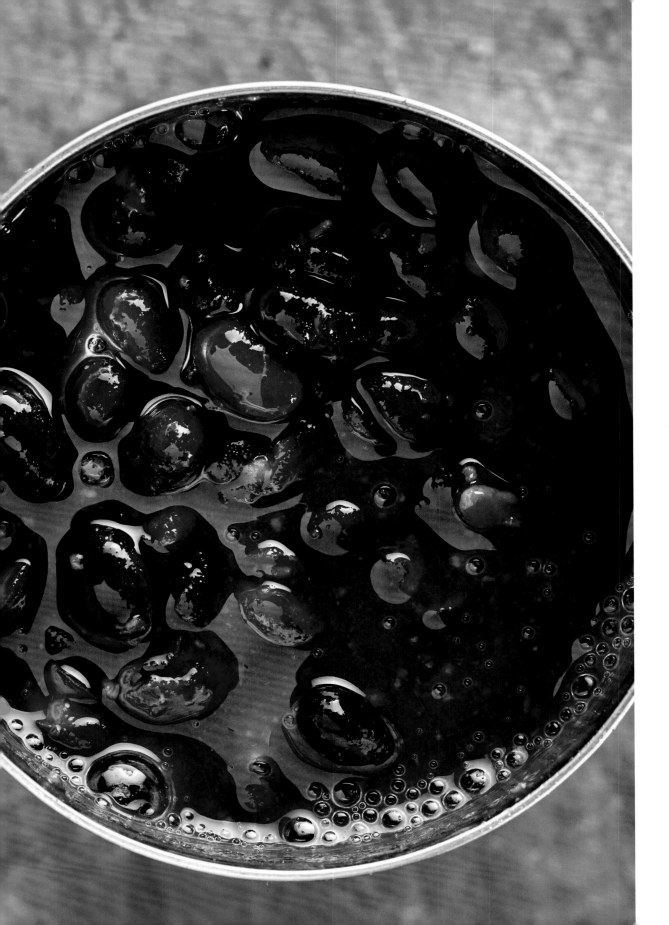

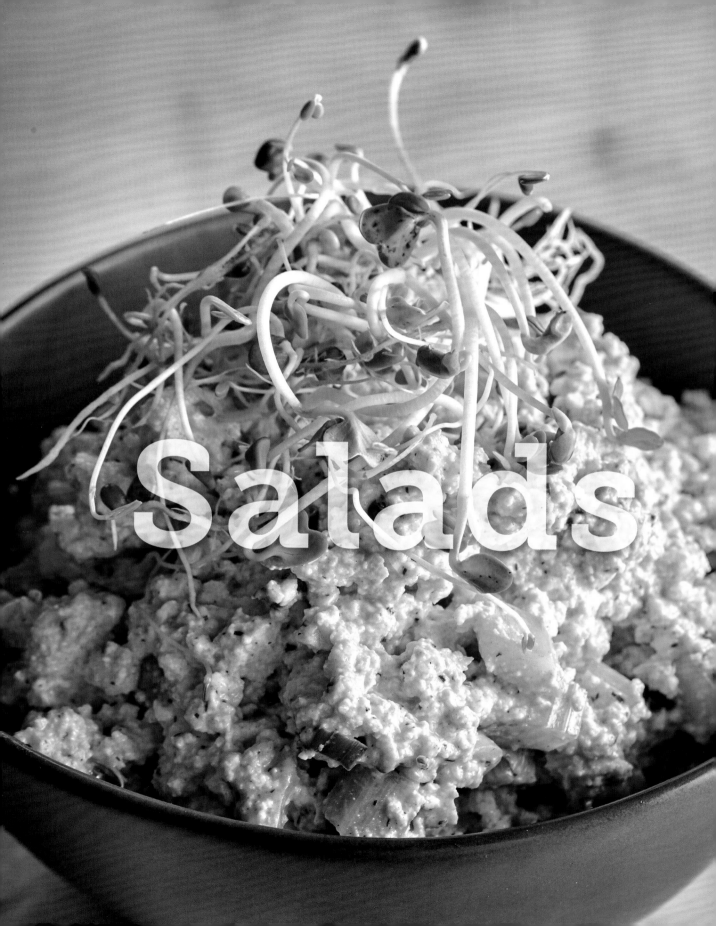

Salads

Salads are versatile and as easy to prepare as a bowl of crisp greens tossed with vinaigrette, or they can be more complex affairs with mixed greens, fruits, nuts, and croutons. Composed salads with edamame, apples, and beans or grains make a beautiful side dish, while chickpea and tofu salads can be turned into a sandwich filling or scooped onto a plate or into a bowl for a salad-plate entree. Dress salads lightly to avoid an abundance of dressing floating around in the bottom of the bowl. This enhances and brightens the salad and allows the flavor of the ingredients to shine through.

❧ Recipes

Skillet Croutons

Sweet and Spicy Chickpea Salad

Tofu Eggless Salad

Warm White Bean Salad

Kale Salad with Ginger-Sesame Vinaigrette

Blueberry Lemon Quinoa Salad

Carrot Golden Raisin Salad

Napa Cabbage Slaw with Sriracha Peanut Sauce

Mediterranean Salad

Apple and Celery Salad with Tahini Dressing

Bean Salad with Lime Vinaigrette

Spring Roll Salad with Sweet Chile Vinaigrette

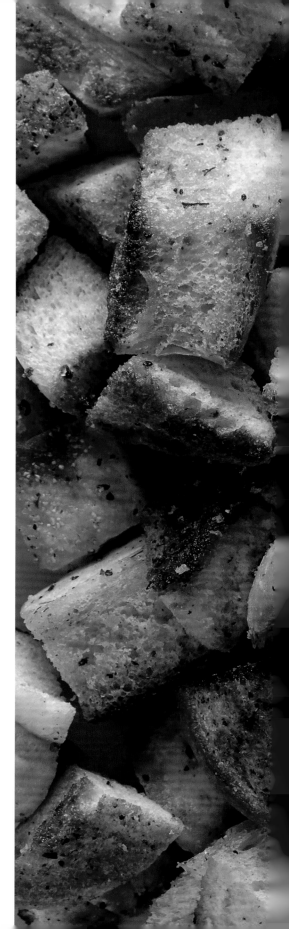

Keeping Salad Greens Fresh

When I buy a plastic "clamshell," or
box, of spring greens, baby spinach, or
baby kale, I frequently see moisture in
the box. Moisture is death to tender
greens, causing slime and leaf decay.
To maintain the freshness of the green,
I open the box and place a single paper
towel on top of the greens closed inside
the box, which works wonders to absorb
moisture and help keep the greens
fresh. Another trick for freshness,
after inserting the paper towel, is to
flip the box and store the paper-towel-
topped box of greens upside down.
Any moisture on the lid is absorbed
and any moisture on the greens flows
toward the absorbent paper towel so
the greens don't sit in the moisture.

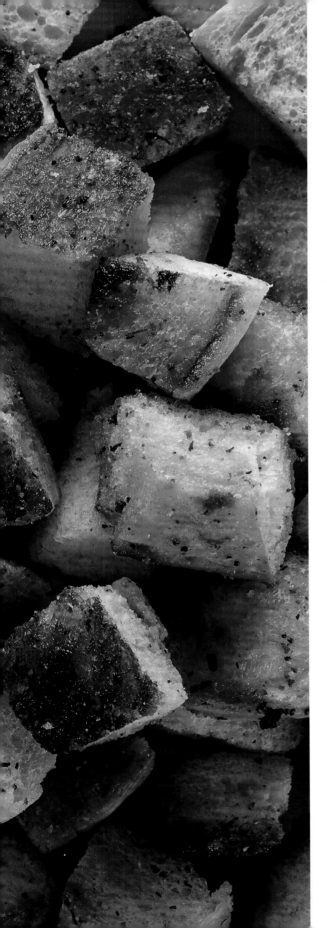

Skillet Croutons

Makes 2 cups

Croutons are a joy to make and even better to eat. They are an excellent way to use day-old bread. While we generally think of croutons made with cubes of bread, croutons can also be made from slices of bread, for a flat crouton or "crostini." To me, taking time to make croutons elevates the dish more than its ready-to-eat counterpart. Bread can be cut ahead of time to dry out a bit if desired. This is also a good use for day-old bread.

Ingredients:

2 cups bread cubes (from about 4 slices bread)
4 tablespoons olive oil, divided
½ teaspoon dried thyme
½ teaspoon kosher salt
½ teaspoon freshly ground black pepper

Directions:

In a bowl, toss the bread cubes with 2 tablespoons olive oil, thyme, salt, and pepper. In a skillet, heat the remaining 2 tablespoons olive oil over medium heat. Add the seasoned bread cubes to the skillet and cook, stirring occasionally for 10 to 12 minutes until the croutons are golden brown. Remove to a plate after cooking so they don't burn.

gluten free

Sweet and Spicy Curried Chickpea Salad

Serves 2

Refreshingly sweet and spicy, this chickpea salad is good on toasted whole-grain bread or on a bed of fresh baby spinach or salad greens. You may add ¼ cup of either Plant-Based Mayonnaise, page 48, if desired, for a more creamy salad. Save the chickpea liquid to make a batch of Plant-Based Mayonnaise 1.

Ingredients:

One 15-ounce can chickpeas, drained,
    or 1 ½ cups cooked chickpeas

½ cup golden raisins

2 tablespoons olive oil

1 tablespoon brown sugar

1 teaspoon curry powder

⅛ teaspoon cayenne pepper

2 tablespoons chopped fresh mint

2 tablespoons chopped fresh cilantro

¼ teaspoon kosher salt

Freshly ground black pepper

Directions:

In a bowl mix the chickpeas, raisins, olive oil, brown sugar, curry powder, cayenne pepper, mint, cilantro, salt, and pepper. Serve at room temperature. Store in the refrigerator.

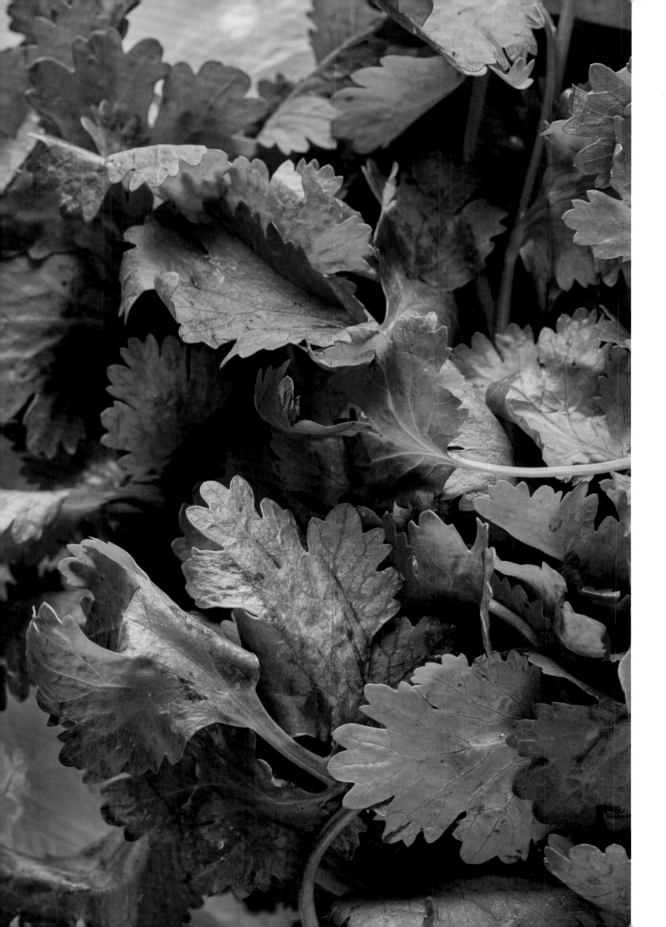

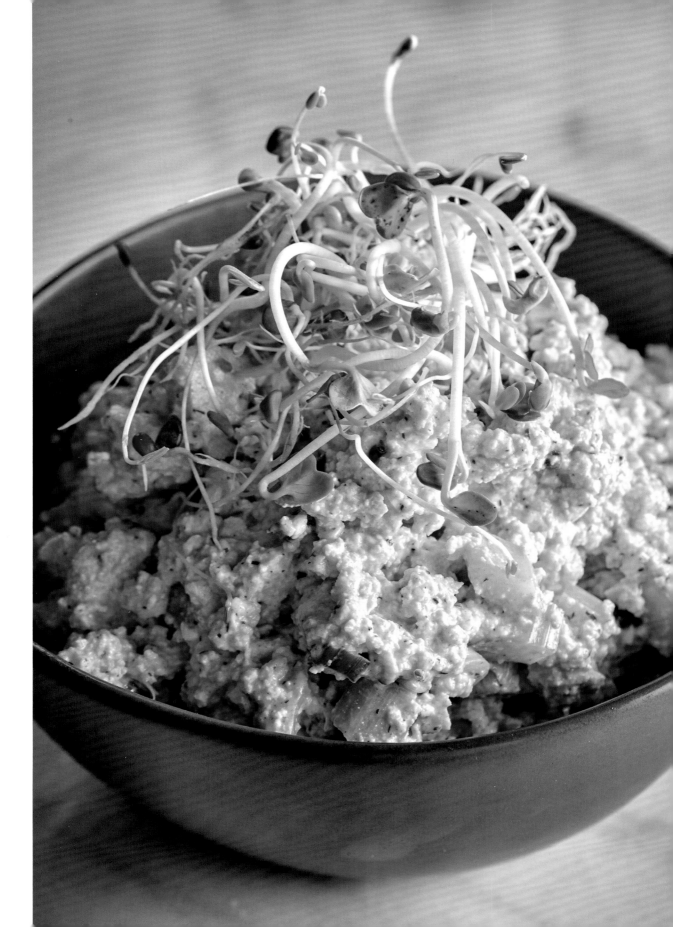

the essential plant-based pantry

Tofu Eggless Salad

Makes about 2 ½ cups

Scoop this eggless salad onto whole-grain or gluten-free bread, or serve it on a bed of fresh lettuce or baby spinach. You will need either Plant-Based Mayonnaise, page 48, for this salad, or you may choose to use another plant-based mayonnaise of your choice, with readily available egg-free commercial mayonnaise.

Ingredients:

One 14-ounce box extra-firm tofu, drained

2 ribs celery, finely chopped

2 green onions, thinly sliced

½ cup Plant-Based Mayonnaise

2 teaspoons Dijon mustard

½ teaspoon ground turmeric

¼ teaspoon dill weed

½ teaspoon kosher salt

½ teaspoon ground black pepper

Directions:

Crumble the tofu into a fine-mesh strainer. With your hands or a silicone spoon or spatula, press the excess moisture out of the crumbled tofu. Let drain in the strainer while you prepare the other ingredients.

In a bowl, combine the celery, green onion, "mayonnaise," mustard, turmeric, dill weed, salt, and pepper. Mix well. Add the crumbled tofu and stir well to combine. Serve immediately or store, covered, in the refrigerator.

Tips for Tossing Salads

I like to use a two-stage approach to add vinaigrette to a salad so that the heavy ingredients don't sink to the bottom of the bowl. To do this first place the greens on the serving platter or in a serving bowl. Drizzle the greens with half of the vinaigrette and toss gently. Then, scatter the toppings over the greens, but don't toss them in. Drizzle with remaining vinaigrette. Now, your greens are dressed and your toppings are on top where they belong!

gluten free

Warm White Bean Salad

Serves 2 to 3

Warm white beans pair beautifully with lemon zest, fresh tomatoes, and mint for a simple entrée or side salad. You can't go wrong if you serve this bean salad with warm or grilled whole-grain bread and a variety of olives.

Ingredients:

One 15-ounce can great northern beans, drained, or 1 ½ cups cooked beans

4 tablespoons olive oil, divided

½ small red onion, thinly sliced

1 cup chopped fresh tomato

Zest of 1 lemon

2 tablespoons lemon juice (from about 1 lemon)

3 cloves garlic, minced

¼ teaspoon kosher salt

Freshly ground black pepper

¼ cup chopped fresh mint

Directions:

Drain beans in a colander and rinse well.

In a saucepan, heat 2 tablespoons olive oil over medium heat. Add the red onion and cook for 6 minutes until softened and starting to brown. Stir in the remaining 2 tablespoons olive oil, tomato, lemon zest, lemon juice, garlic, salt, and pepper. Reduce heat to low and cook gently for about 5 minutes to soften the garlic and tomatoes and blend the flavors.

Remove from the heat and fold in the beans and fresh mint. Move to a serving bowl and serve warm or at room temperature.

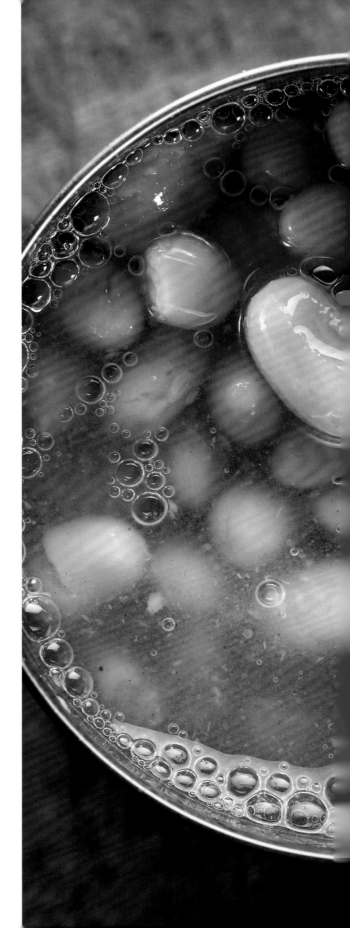

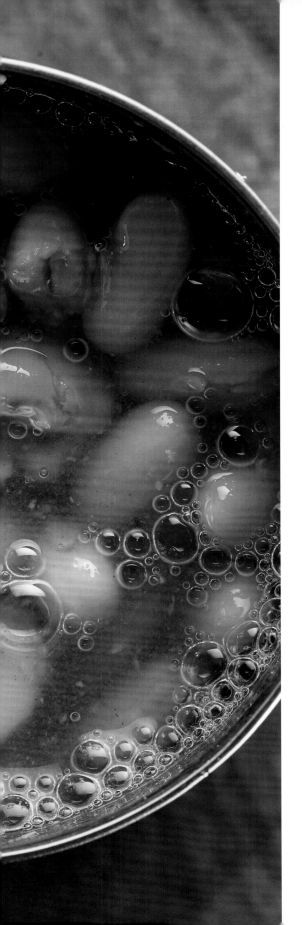

Tamari

Tamari is a thick brown sauce made from soybeans. Generally wheat free, though not always, tamari has very few ingredients. It can be used in place of soy sauce in recipes. This is my sauce of choice in recipe where soy sauce is used.

Massaged Kale

Learning how to massage kale, and more importantly why to massage kale, changed the way I feel about kale salads. Fresh kale can be tough and hard to chew and digest. Rubbing olive oil and salt into the chopped kale leaves softens them, breaks down the tough fibers, and turns the kale a beautiful deep green color. To prepare the kale for massaging, rinse and dry the kale leaves. Remove the tough stems and cut the kale into bite-sized pieces. Place the kale leaves in a bowl, and rub the olive oil and salt into the leaves for about one to two minutes. Let the leaves sit while preparing the other ingredients.

Kale Salad with Ginger-Sesame Vinaigrette

gluten free

Serves 4

Massage the cleaned and chopped kale with olive oil and salt to soften the kale and prepare it for this beautiful kale salad. This step of massaging is transformative to the kale, and you and your kale salads will never be the same! Alternatively, if you're not into massaging kale, you can substitute six cups of baby kale or baby spinach.

Salad ingredients:

1 large bunch green or purple kale

1 tablespoon olive oil

½ teaspoon kosher salt

1 cucumber, peeled

1 cup chopped red cabbage

½ cup dried cranberries

¼ cup almond slices, toasted

Ginger sesame vinaigrette ingredients:

2 tablespoons canola oil

1 tablespoon toasted sesame oil

1 tablespoon apple cider vinegar

1 tablespoon honey

1 tablespoon fresh grated ginger root
   or ginger paste

2 cloves garlic, peeled and minced

1 teaspoon reduced-sodium soy sauce or tamari

¼ teaspoon freshly ground black pepper

Directions:

Remove stems from the kale. Wash leaves well and spin to dry or roll them in a clean kitchen towel to absorb excess water. Stack the clean leaves and tightly roll into a long tube. With a sharp knife, cut the leaves into thin slices. Place in a bowl and sprinkle with olive oil and salt. With your hands, massage the oil and salt into the kale leaves for about 1 minute. Let sit while you prepare other ingredients and the vinaigrette.

Slice the cucumber in half and scrape out the seeds with a spoon. Cut into slices.

To make the vinaigrette, combine all ingredients in a blender or shake well in a jar.

Place kale in a shallow serving bowl or platter. Toss with half of the vinaigrette. Top with cucumber, red cabbage, dried cranberries, and almond slices. Drizzle with remaining Ginger Sesame Vinaigrette and serve.

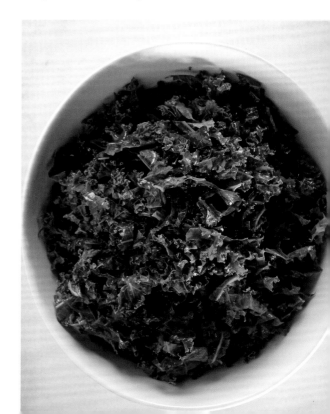

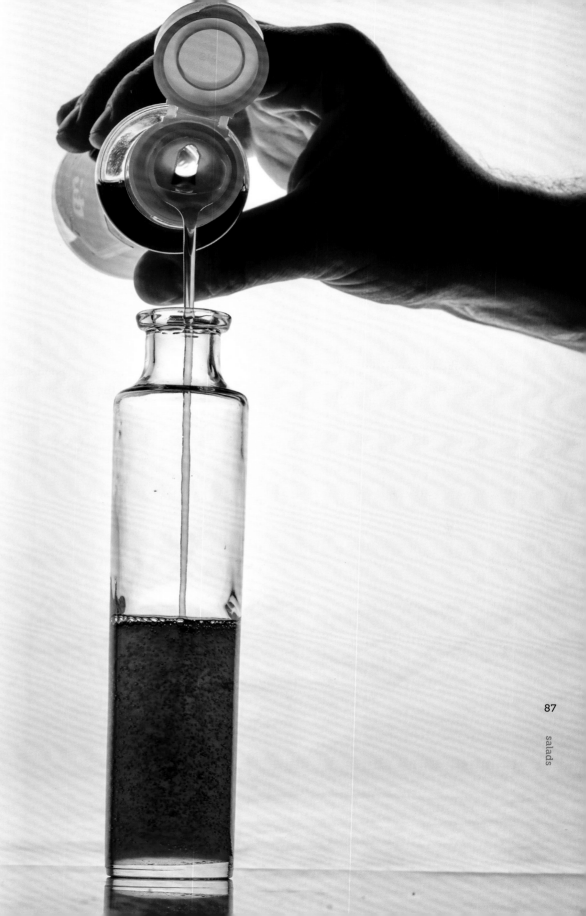

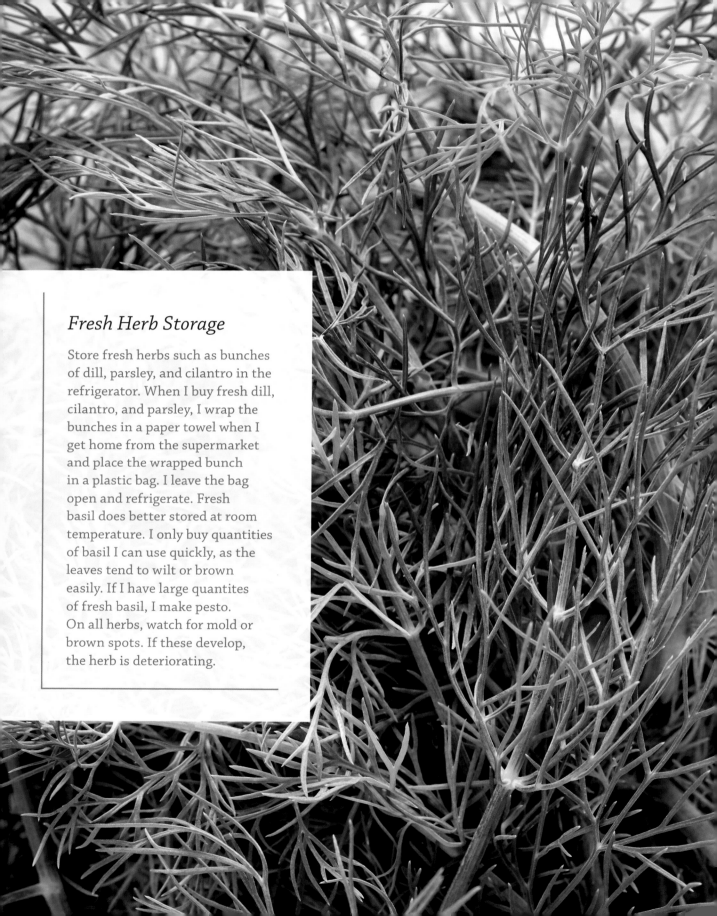

Fresh Herb Storage

Store fresh herbs such as bunches of dill, parsley, and cilantro in the refrigerator. When I buy fresh dill, cilantro, and parsley, I wrap the bunches in a paper towel when I get home from the supermarket and place the wrapped bunch in a plastic bag. I leave the bag open and refrigerate. Fresh basil does better stored at room temperature. I only buy quantities of basil I can use quickly, as the leaves tend to wilt or brown easily. If I have large quantites of fresh basil, I make pesto. On all herbs, watch for mold or brown spots. If these develop, the herb is deteriorating.

Blueberry Lemon Quinoa Salad

Serves 4

For best results, toss the salad with the vinaigrette just before serving. One cup of any cooked grain, such as brown rice, can be used in place of the quinoa.

Ingredients:

½ cup uncooked quinoa

1 cup water

1 cup fresh blueberries

2 cups baby arugula

2 tablespoons lemon juice (from about 1 lemon)

1 teaspoon Dijon mustard

1 tablespoon honey

4 tablespoons olive oil

½ teaspoon kosher salt

¼ teaspoon freshly ground black pepper

Directions:

To prepare quinoa, place dry/uncooked quinoa in a fine mesh strainer. Rinse under cold water for 1 minute to remove a coating on the quinoa that can cause stomach upset or bitterness. Place the rinsed quinoa in a small saucepan and add 1 cup water. Over medium heat, bring to a boil. Reduce heat to low and simmer uncovered until the water is absorbed, about 10 minutes. Remove from heat and cover. Let sit for 5 minutes. Fluff with a fork and move to a plate to cool.

Meanwhile, wash the blueberries and thinly slice the arugula. In a serving bowl whisk together the lemon juice, mustard, honey, olive oil, salt, and pepper. Gently fold in the cooled quinoa, blueberries, and arugula.

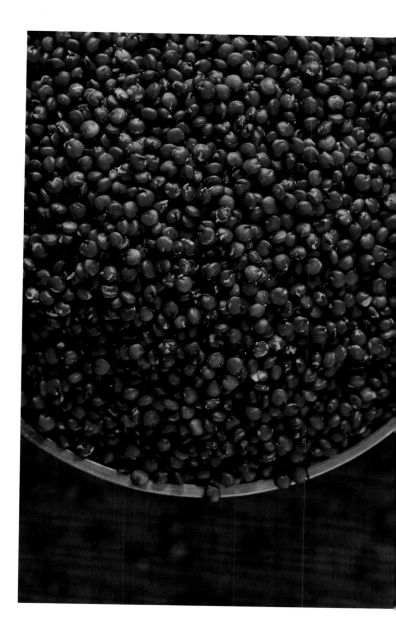

89

salads

gluten free

Carrot Golden Raisin Salad

Serves 6 to 8

Create a high-protein twist on carrot raisin salad: add green soybeans, or edamame. Then dress the vegetables with a light lemon vinaigrette instead of mayonnaise. Edamame is sold frozen in the pod, or out of the pod. For this recipe, you want to use the shelled (out of the pod) edamame.

Ingredients:

1 ¼ cups frozen shelled edamame

½ cup sliced almonds

2 tablespoons lemon juice (from about 1 lemon)

1 teaspoon Dijon mustard

1 tablespoon honey

4 tablespoons olive oil

½ teaspoon cumin

½ teaspoon kosher salt

¼ teaspoon freshly ground black pepper

2 carrots, peeled and shredded

¼ cup flat-leaf parsley

¾ cup golden raisins

Directions:

Place edamame in a microwave-safe dish or small saucepan. Add ½ inch of water and cover. Either cook in a microwave oven on high power for 5 minutes, or bring to a boil, reduce heat to a simmer, and cook for 5 minutes. Drain before using.

In a small skillet, toast the almonds over low heat. Remove to a plate to cool.

Meanwhile, in a bowl whisk together the lemon juice, mustard, honey, olive oil, cumin, salt, and pepper. Fold in the carrots, parsley, raisins, and cooled edamame. Top with sliced, toasted almonds and serve.

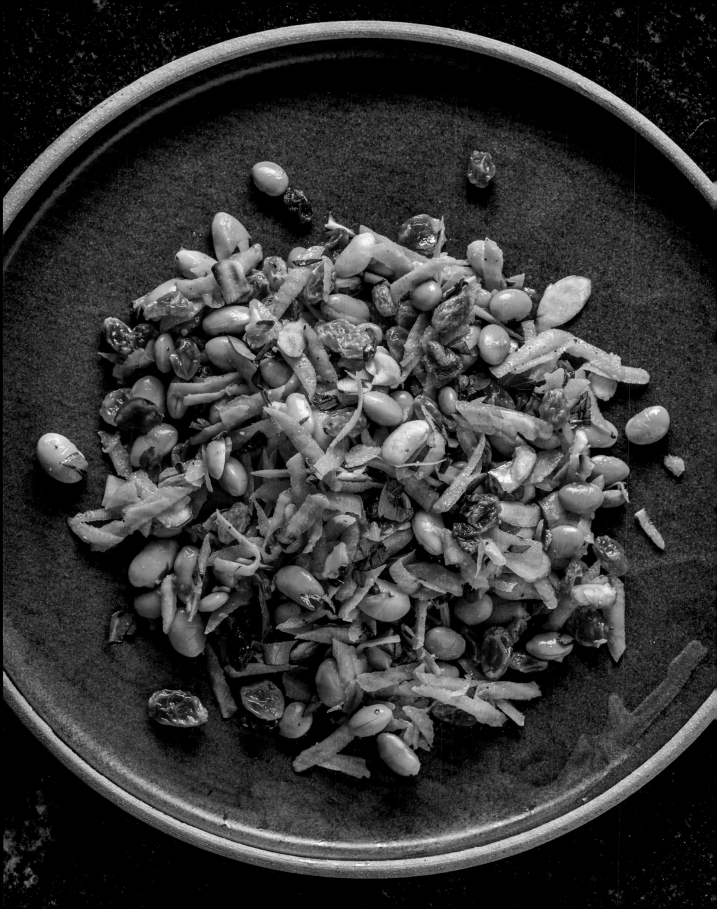

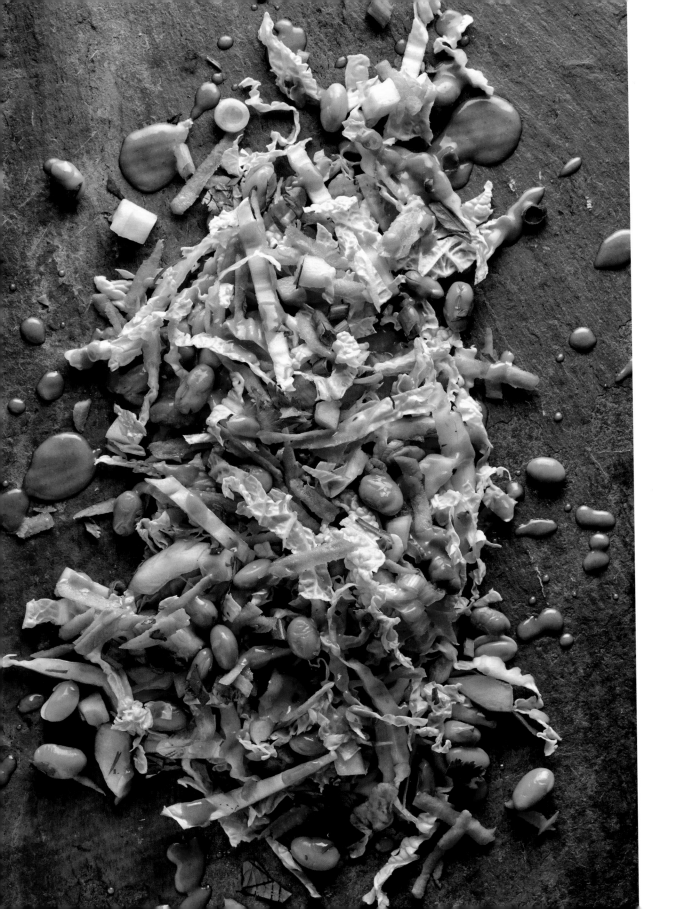

Napa Cabbage Slaw with Sriracha Peanut Sauce

Makes 6 cups

Napa cabbage has beautiful crinkly leaves and a mild flavor. Three cups of green or red cabbage, or slaw mix, can be substituted.

Ingredients:

1 cup frozen shelled edamame

3 cups thinly sliced napa cabbage

1 cucumber, peeled, halved, seeded, and cut into half moons

1 carrot, peeled and grated

2 green onions, thinly sliced

½ cup chopped fresh parsley, cilantro, mint, or basil

Optional: ½ cup sliced almonds, toasted

Sriracha Peanut Sauce, page 55

Directions:

Place edamame in a microwave-safe dish or small saucepan. Add ½ inch of water and cover. Either cook in a microwave oven on high power for 5 minutes, or bring to a boil, reduce heat to a simmer, and cook for 5 minutes. Drain before using.

In a bowl, mix the cooled edamame, cabbage, cucumber, carrot, green onion, cilantro, and optional almonds.

Mix half of the peanut sauce into the prepared vegetables. Toss to blend with the dressing. Add more if desired.

Fresh Herbs

If you want to elevate your cooking, use fresh herbs to finish a dish. Parsley, cilantro, basil, rosemary, and mint can't be beat when finely chopped and used to finish a dish. I rarely use fresh herbs while cooking a dish. In cooking, dried thyme, oregano, dill, and basil work just fine.

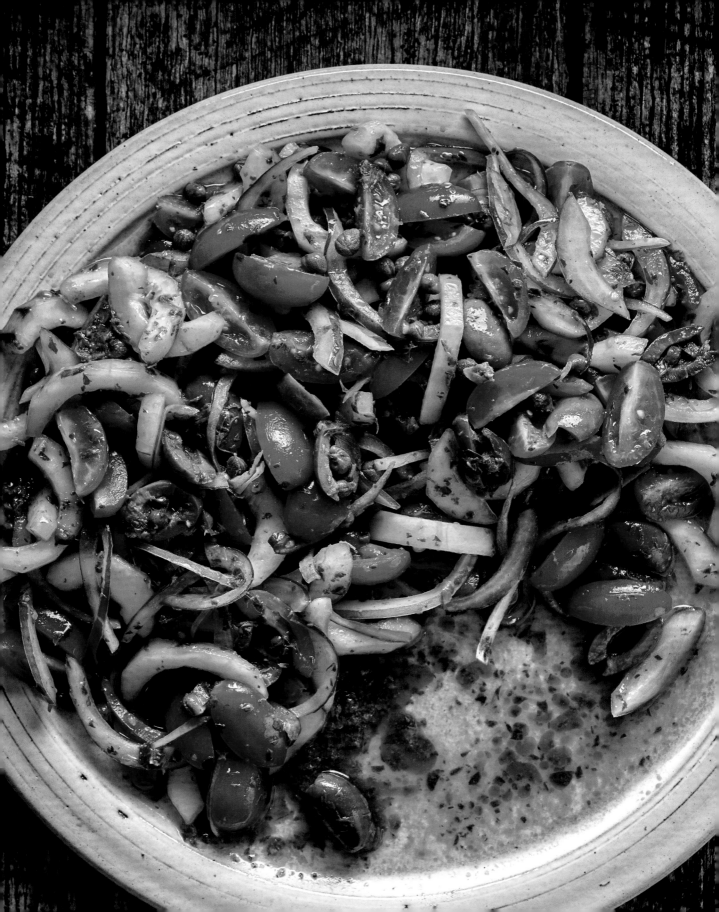

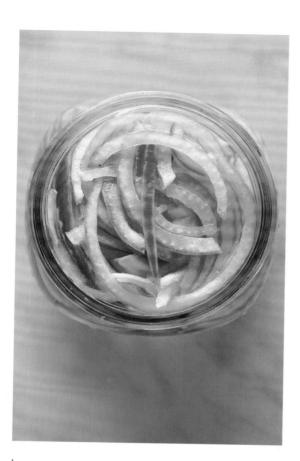

Mediterranean Salad

gluten free

Serves 4

This fresh salad with a beautiful green herb vinaigrette makes a nice accompaniment to Barbecue Lentils, page 126, or Kidney Bean Burgers, page 148. It can be prepared ahead and refrigerated until served.

Ingredients:

1 cucumber, peeled, seeded, and sliced

1 cup grape tomatoes, quartered

1 cup pitted Kalamata olives

½ medium red onion, thinly sliced
   and soaked in water

¼ cup capers

⅓ cup Fresh Herb Vinaigrette, page 52

Directions:

In a bowl mix together the cucumber, tomatoes, olives, red onion, and capers. Mix in the vinaigrette and serve.

Soaking Red Onion

There's no doubt that on salads and sandwiches, red onion's color adds appeal. Red onion, on the other hand, can have a very sharp, oniony taste that lingers. When I use red onion in salads, I soak raw slices in water for fifteen minutes before adding it to salads, or I pickle a jar of red onions to have on hand. Here's my super-easy pickled onion recipe: page 18.

Apple and Celery Salad with Tahini Dressing

gluten free

Serves 4

This spin on Waldorf salad is made egg-free and more modern with a creamy tahini dressing, and walnuts, capers, and golden raisins. Toss the apples with the dressing just before serving to prevent the apples from browning.

Ingredients:

2 Golden Delicious apples, cored and thinly sliced

3 ribs celery, thinly sliced on the diagonal

2 tablespoons tahini

1 tablespoon olive oil

2 tablespoons lemon juice (from about 1 lemon)

2 tablespoons water

⅛ teaspoon kosher salt

¼ teaspoon freshly ground black pepper

¼ cup chopped walnuts

2 tablespoons capers

2 tablespoons golden raisins

Directions:

Mix together the apples and celery in a bowl. Whisk together the tahini, olive oil, lemon juice, salt, and pepper. Combine the dressing with the apples and celery. Stir in the walnuts, capers, and raisins. Serve pretty soon after mixing in the dressing, because the apples may turn brown if left exposed to air too long.

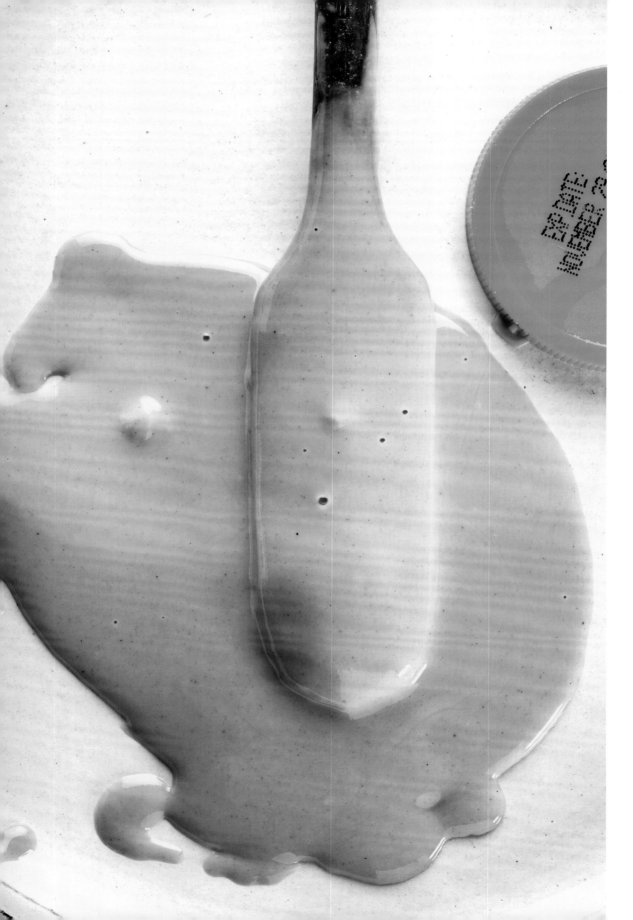

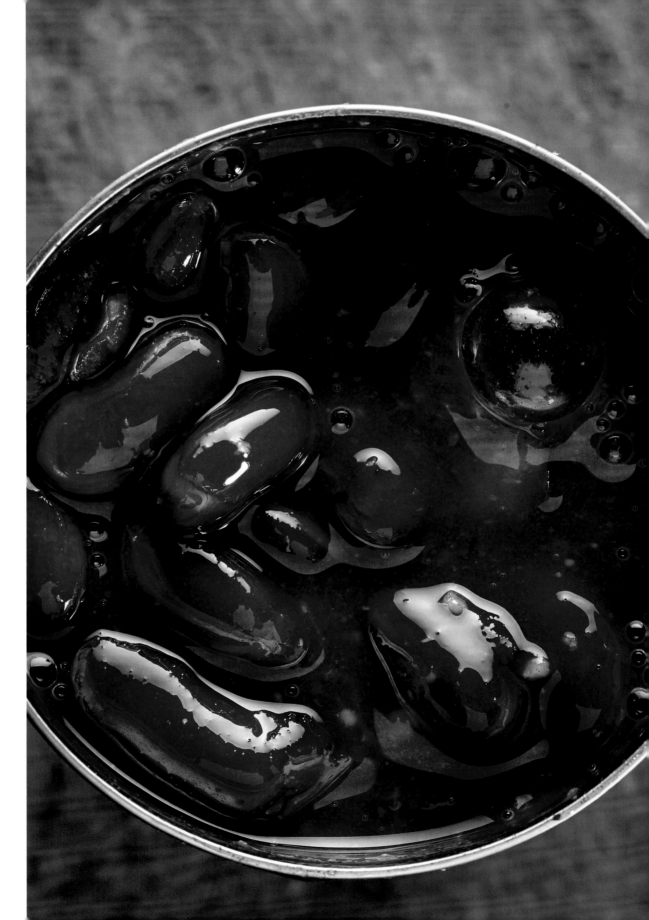

the essential plant-based pantry

Bean Salad with Lime Vinaigrette gluten free

Serves 4 to 6

This is a nice salad to make with leftover rice, wheat berries, or quinoa. If you need to cook the grain, start with ⅔ cup of uncooked rice or quinoa or one cup uncooked wheat berries to yield two cups of cooked grain for the salad. For best results, add the dressing just before serving the salad.

Ingredients:

¼ cup finely diced red onion, soaked in water

One 15-ounce can black beans, drained and rinsed, or 1 ½ cups cooked black beans

One 15-ounce can red, or kidney beans drained and rinsed, or 1 ½ cups cooked red or kidney beans

2 cups cooked brown rice, wheat berries, or quinoa

½ cup diced roasted red pepper

½ cup fresh cilantro

¼ cup olive oil

¼ cup fresh lime juice (from about 2 limes)

2 tablespoons honey

1 clove garlic, peeled and minced

1 teaspoon smoked paprika

¾ teaspoon cumin

¾ teaspoon kosher salt

¼ teaspoon freshly ground black pepper

Directions:

Soak chopped red onion in a bowl of warm water.

In a serving bowl, mix the beans, cooked rice or wheat berries, roasted red pepper, and cilantro.

In a small bowl whisk together the olive oil, lime juice, honey, garlic, smoked paprika, cumin, salt, and pepper.

Combine the dressing with the bean mixture. Drain and add the red onion. Serve at room temperature.

Spring Roll Salad with Sweet Chile Vinaigrette

Serves 6

This fresh salad contains ingredients found in Vietnamese spring rolls. The greens and vegetables are tossed with a sweet vinaigrette that is similar to a spring roll dipping sauce. The trio of fresh herbs make the salad complete, but if desired, you can use only cilantro and/or basil depending on the availability of mint and other herbs. For a hit of protein, add Pan-Fried Tofu, page 157.

For best results, toss the lettuce and herbs with the vinaigrette just before serving. I like to arrange the remaining "heavy" vegetables, such as red pepper, cucumber, and carrot, on top of the dressed greens and drizzle them with vinaigrette. If the "heavy" vegetables are tossed in with the greens, they invariably sink to the bottom of the bowl.

Fresh ginger makes all the difference here. Use either peeled and grated fresh ginger root, or fresh ground ginger paste sold in tubes or small bottles in the produce section.

Salad ingredients:

1 romaine heart or small head Butter or
　Bibb Lettuce, cleaned and torn into
　1-inch pieces (about 4 cups)

1 red pepper, seeded and thinly sliced

2 carrots, peeled and thinly sliced or
　cut into strips

1 cucumber, peeled, seeded, and thinly sliced

1 cup fresh cilantro leaves

½ cup fresh mint, chopped

½ cup fresh basil, chopped

Optional: fresh mung bean sprouts

Optional: Pan-Fried Tofu

Sweet chile vinaigrette ingredients:

¼ cup water

2 tablespoons apple cider vinegar

2 tablespoons honey

1 tablespoon olive oil

2 tablespoons lime juice
　(from about 1–2 limes)

1 tablespoon fresh grated ginger root or
　ginger paste

2 cloves garlic, minced

½ teaspoon red pepper flakes

1 teaspoon sriracha

Directions:

Have all salad ingredients ready.

In a small bowl, combine the water, vinegar, and honey. Whisk just to combine and dissolve the honey. Whisk in the oil, lime juice, ginger, garlic, red pepper flakes, and sriracha, and combine until well blended.

On a platter or in a bowl, place the lettuce. Drizzle with half of the vinaigrette and toss. Mix in the herbs and a bit more vinaigrette and toss. Top with red pepper, carrot, and cucumber, but don't toss. Drizzle with remaining vinaigrette. Top with optional mung bean sprouts or Pan-Fried Tofu if desired.

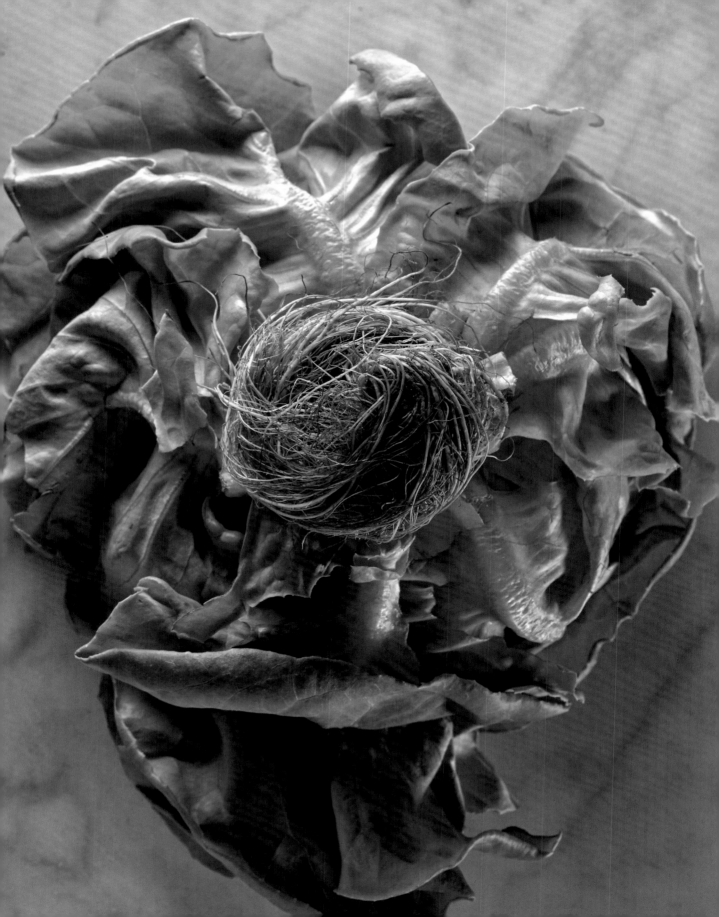

Sides

It's often said that the side dishes make the meal. And I think I agree. How can you go wrong when you start with vegetables, grains, and pasta; add spices, herbs, nuts, and seasoning; and end up with a side dish that adds color and texture to a meal? I enjoy the seasonal variety a side dish can add to a meal. Sometimes, we make a meal out of several side dishes where everyone takes a scoop of each and creates their own vegetable plate supper.

❧ Recipes

Mac and No Cheese

Sweet Potato and Onion Hash Browns

Sesame Honey Brussels Sprouts

Spiced Rice Pilaf with Golden Raisins and Almonds

Braised Eggplant and Lemon

Roasted Cauliflower with Almond Curry Pesto

Roasted Cardamom Carrots

Edamame Succotash

Foil-Roasted Parsnips and Carrots

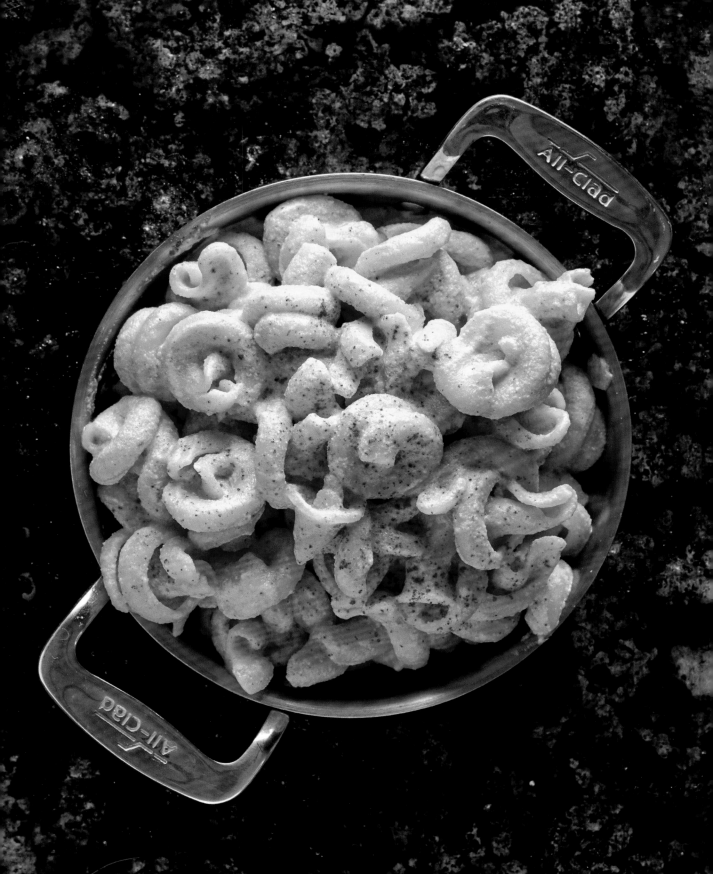

Mac and No Cheese

Serves 6

Twirly or tube-shaped pasta, such as macaroni or penne, works best in this recipe to catch the creamy sauce. Allow at least four hours to soak the cashews for the best results. If you plan to make this for supper, soak the cashews in the morning while you're making your coffee, and then you'll be all set when the dinner bell rings. I have made this without soaking the cashews, and the results are not as creamy—you end up with little pieces of cashew in the sauce. See more about raw cashews, page 38.

Ingredients:

1 cup raw cashews

2 cups water, plus more for soaking

2 cups rotini or other twirly pasta

1 teaspoon Dijon mustard

1 teaspoon ground turmeric

1 teaspoon onion powder

⅛ teaspoon cayenne pepper

¾ teaspoon kosher salt

Directions:

Place raw cashews in a glass or other heat-proof bowl. Cover with 1 inch of hot water. Cover the bowl and soak overnight or at least 8 hours. This softens the cashews to make them easy to blend.

After the cashews have soaked, proceed with cooking the pasta and making the sauce.

In a large pot of boiling water, cook the rotini for about 9 to 11 minutes or until just tender. Drain in a colander, rinse with hot water, and return to the pan. Some may argue that rinsing the pasta removes the starch from the pasta surface—in this case that's true and is desirable. If not rinsed, it may be hard to mix in the cashew cream sauce.

To make the cashew cream, drain the cashew soaking water. Using a blender, mix the cashews and 2 cups water on high speed for 2 minutes. Scrape down the sides and and process again until smooth and creamy. Add the mustard, turmeric, onion powder, cayenne pepper, and salt. Process again to mix well. Add the sauce to the pasta and stir to coat well. Turn the heat to medium-low to gently heat the pasta and the sauce.

Sweet Potato and Onion Hash Browns

Serves 4

A simple way to cook and serve sweet potatoes, this recipe is even better when topped with Almond Curry Pesto, page 43, or Olive Spread, page 21.

Ingredients:

2 tablespoons olive oil

1 medium onion, peeled and
   very thinly sliced

1 pound sweet potatoes, peeled and
   grated (about 2 cups shredded)

½ teaspoon kosher salt

½ teaspoon freshly ground black pepper

Directions:

In a large skillet, heat olive oil over medium-high heat. Add the onion and cook until light golden brown, about 8 minutes. Put the grated potatoes in the skillet and pat the potatoes down to compact them. Let cook for about 5 to 7 minutes, without stirring, until golden brown on the bottom. Flip the potatoes with a spatula and press them down. Cook for about 5 more minutes until golden brown. Stir and season with salt and pepper. Serve hot.

Sesame Honey Brussels Sprouts

Serves 4

Take one large, hot skillet and some fresh Brussels sprouts, and in a few minutes you have a nice, spicy side dish.

Ingredients:

2 tablespoons canola or olive oil

1 pound Brussels sprouts, trimmed and
   halved from stem to top

4 cloves garlic, peeled and minced

3 tablespoons honey

1 tablespoon red wine vinegar

1 tablespoon toasted sesame oil

¾ teaspoon kosher salt

⅛ to ¼ teaspoon red pepper flakes,
   depending on how spicy you want
   the sprouts

Directions:

Heat canola or olive oil in a large skillet over medium heat. Add the halved Brussels sprouts and toss in the oil. With a spatula, press the Brussels sprouts into a single layer. Cover and let cook on medium heat for 2 minutes. Uncover and shake the pan to move the Brussels sprouts around, press into a single layer, cover, and cook for 2 more minutes. Add the garlic and stir well. Cook for just a few minutes until the garlic is fragrant.

In a small bowl, whisk together the honey, red wine vinegar, sesame oil, salt, and your preferred quantity of red pepper flakes.

Add the honey mixture to the Brussels sprouts. Stir well and cook for 1 minute to combine the flavors. Do not overcook. You want to maintain a bright green color and crunchy texture. Remove to a platter and serve warm.

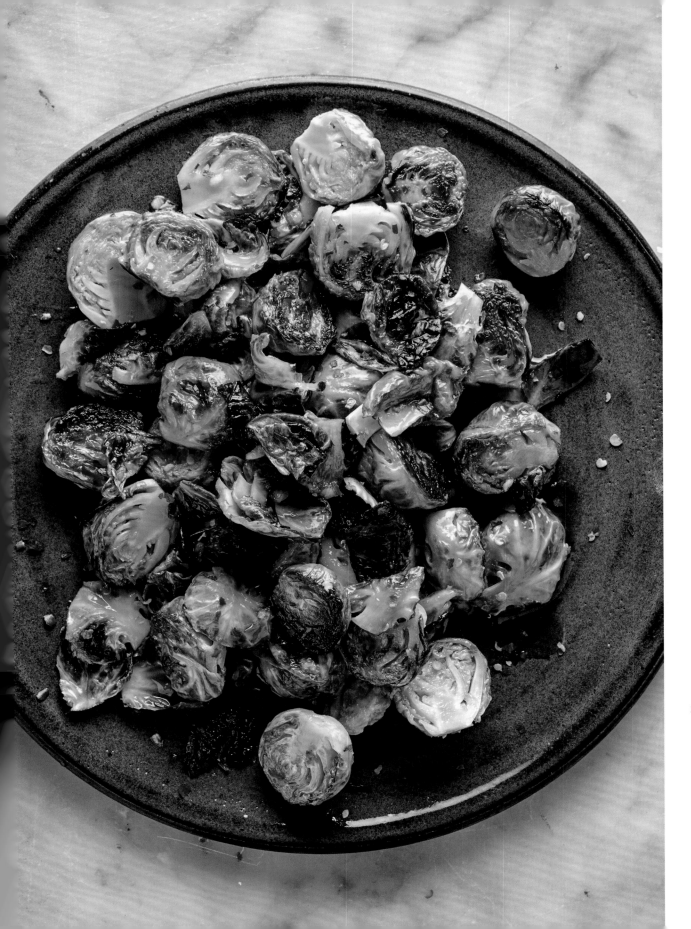

Spiced Rice Pilaf with Golden Raisins and Almonds

gluten free

Serves 6

I love spicy rice pilafs made with black pepper and coriander. The raisins and almonds enhance the dish with sweetness and crunch. Any long-grain white or brown rice works for this recipe, but basmati rice has a fragrance all its own that works beautifully in this pilaf. If you use brown rice, extend the cooking time to forty-five minutes.

Ingredients:

1 tablespoon olive oil

½ small onion, finely chopped (about ¼ cup)

1 cup basmati or other long-grain rice

½ teaspoon coriander

½ teaspoon cardamom

½ teaspoon freshly ground black pepper

¼ teaspoon kosher salt

2 cups water

½ cup sliced almonds

½ cup golden raisins

Directions:

In a saucepan heat the oil over medium heat. Add the onion and cook about 8 minutes until golden. Stir in the rice, coriander, cardamom, black pepper, and salt. Stir to toast the rice for about 1 minute. Add the water and bring to a boil. Stir, cover, reduce the heat to low, and cook for 15 minutes.

Meanwhile, toast the almonds in a small skillet. Remove to a small plate.

When the 15 minutes has elapsed for the rice, turn off the heat, but don't uncover the rice. Let sit, covered, for 10 minutes. When ready to serve, fluff the rice with a fork and top with the golden raisins and toasted almonds.

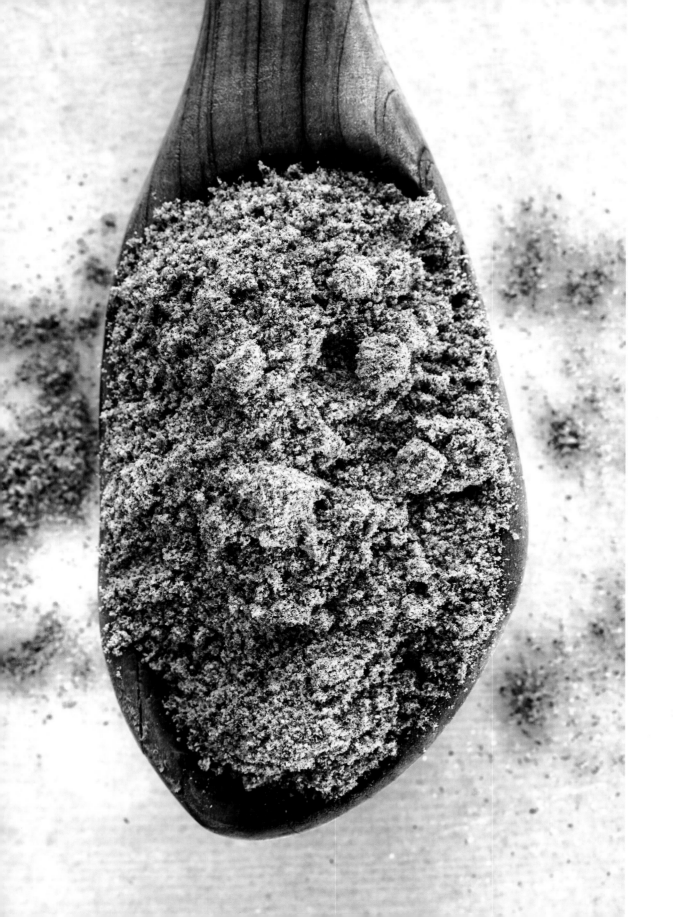

gluten free

Braised Eggplant and Lemon

Serves 8

Eggplant creates a neutral palette for this side dish made with chickpeas, and very thinly sliced lemon. A drizzle of honey or olive oil is nice just before serving. Save the chickpea liquid to make a batch of Plant-Based Mayonnaise 1, page 48.

Ingredients:

1 medium-size globe eggplant

2 tablespoons olive oil

1 medium onion, chopped

6 cloves garlic, sliced

1 small lemon, very thinly sliced

¾ cup chopped roasted red pepper

One 15-ounce can chickpeas, drained, or
    1 ½ cups cooked chickpeas

¾ cup vegetable broth

2 teaspoons smoked paprika

1 teaspoon cumin

1 teaspoon kosher salt

¼ cup chopped fresh basil

Optional: 2 tablespoons honey or olive oil

Directions:

Cut the eggplant in half lengthwise and then into thin ¼-inch, half-circle slices.

Meanwhile, in a large skillet heat olive oil over medium heat. Add the onion and cook until softened and golden about 8 minutes. Add the eggplant slices and cook, stirring occasionally until it is very soft and starts to brown and break apart, about 10 more minutes. Add the garlic, lemon slices, roasted red pepper, chickpeas, vegetable broth, smoked paprika, cumin, and salt.

Bring to a boil, reduce heat and simmer, partially covered, for about 25 minutes until the lemon slices are soft. Stir in the chopped fresh basil. Season to taste with salt and pepper if needed. Serve with a drizzle of honey or olive oil.

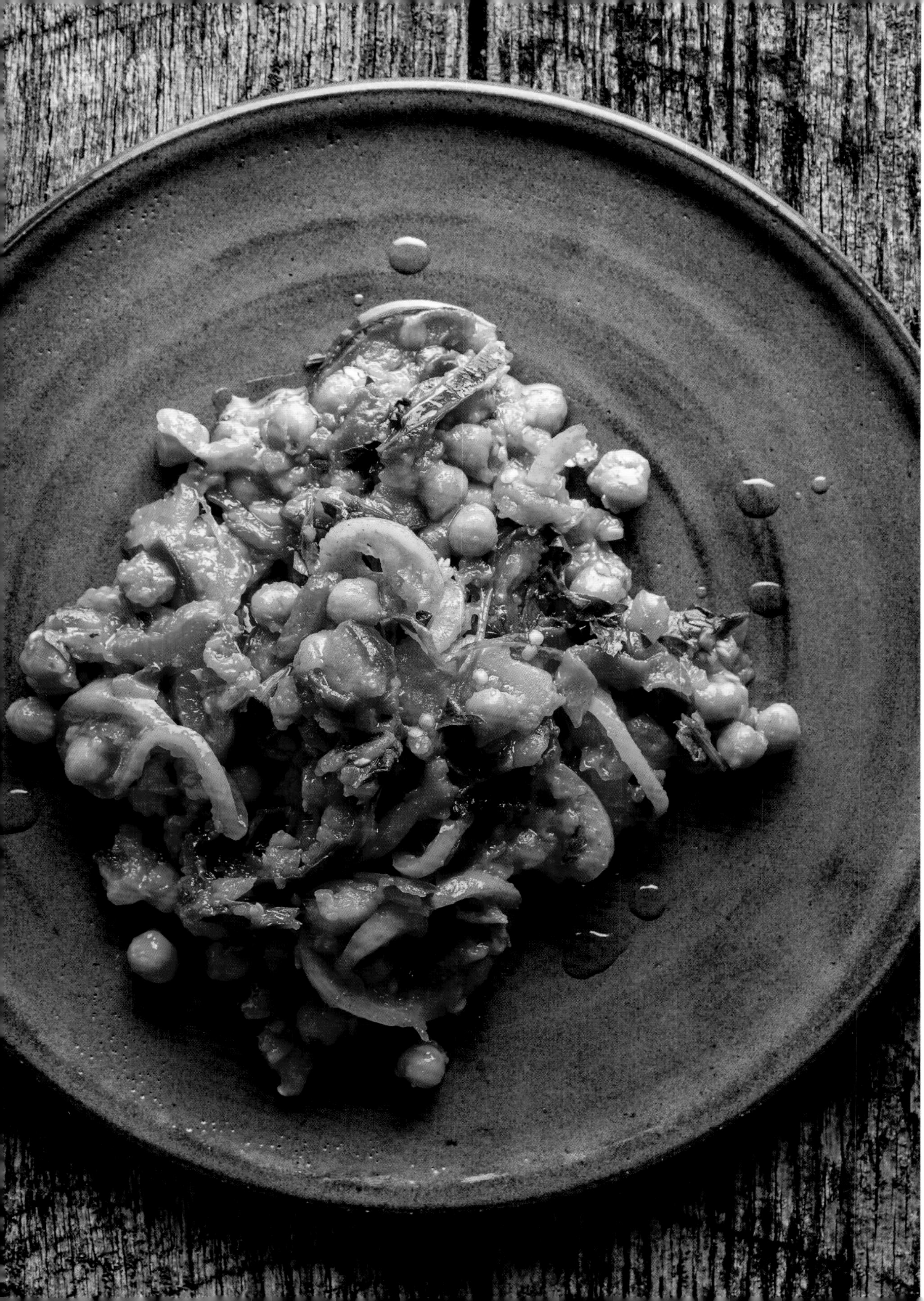

gluten free

Roasted Cauliflower with Almond Curry Pesto

Serves 6

Cauliflower roasted in the oven is a carefree way to prepare it, and the browning that occurs adds color and taste to the vegetable. This is a hearty dish that stores well in the refrigerator after cooking and is good at room temperature as a leftover as well.

Ingredients:

1 medium head cauliflower,
    cut into 2-inch florets

2 tablespoons olive oil

½ teaspoon dried thyme

¼ teaspoon kosher salt

Freshly ground black pepper

Almond Curry Pesto, page 43

Directions:

Preheat oven to 425°F.

    Toss cauliflower with olive oil, thyme, salt, and pepper. Spread in a single layer on a rimmed baking sheet. Bake for 20 minutes or until golden brown. Keep an eye on the cauliflower. The time that this will take depends on the size of the cauliflower pieces. You want it to be browned and tender.

    Meanwhile, prepare the Almond Curry Pesto. Place half of the pesto in a serving bowl. When the cauliflower is roasted, and while it's still warm, spoon the cauliflower into the serving bowl on top of the pesto. Mix gently to coat the cauliflower with the pesto. Serve warm.

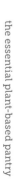

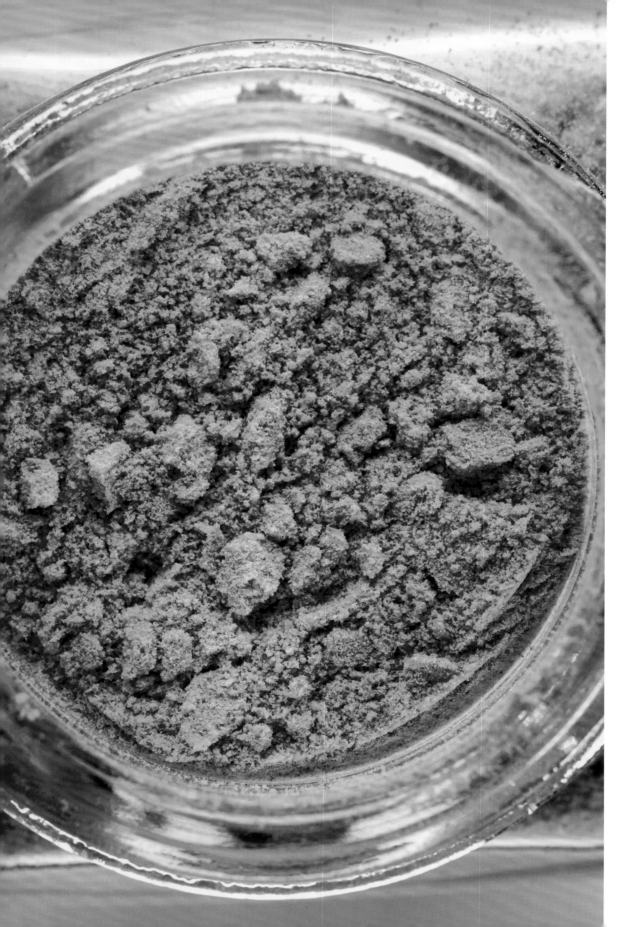

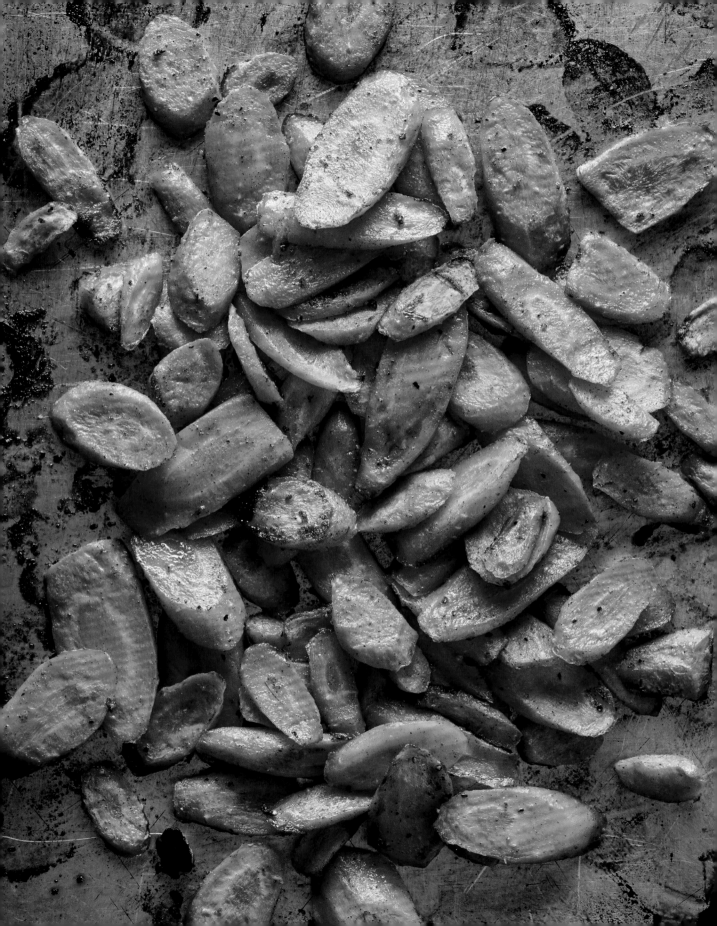

gluten free

Roasted Cardamom Carrots

Serves 4

Simple and spicy, these sweet roasted carrots are a flavorful and colorful side dish that is easy to prepare in the oven while the cook tends to other things.

Ingredients:

8 large carrots, peeled and sliced
  on the diagonal

2 tablespoons olive oil

1 tablespoon honey

¾ teaspoon cardamom

¼ teaspoon kosher salt

¼ teaspoon freshly ground black pepper

Directions:

Preheat oven to 425°F.

Place all ingredients in a bowl and toss to coat carrots with the oil, honey, and spices.

Dump carrots onto a rimmed baking sheet and spread into an even layer.

Roast for 25 to 30 minutes or until carrots are tender and browned.

Edamame Succotash

Serves 4

This side dish substitutes edamame for lima beans, which are traditional in succotash. Add roasted red pepper too for color and flavor.

Ingredients:

1 ½ cups frozen shelled edamame

2 tablespoons olive oil

½ medium onion, diced, or 4 green onions, thinly sliced (about 1 cup)

½ cup chopped roasted red pepper

1 clove garlic, minced

½ teaspoon dried thyme

1 ½ cups fresh or frozen corn kernels (about 3 ears)

½ teaspoon kosher salt

½ teaspoon freshly ground black pepper

Directions:

Place edamame in a microwave-safe dish or small saucepan. Add ½ inch of water and cover. Either cook in a microwave oven on high power for 5 minutes, or bring to a boil, reduce heat to a simmer, and cook for 5 minutes. Drain before using.

In a large skillet, heat olive oil over medium heat. Add the onion and cook for about 6 minutes until the onion is softened and starting to turn golden. Add the red pepper, garlic, and thyme and cook, stirring for 1 to 2 minute until garlic is fragrant. Add the corn, edamame, salt, and pepper. Stir well and let cook for 5 minutes to combine the flavors.

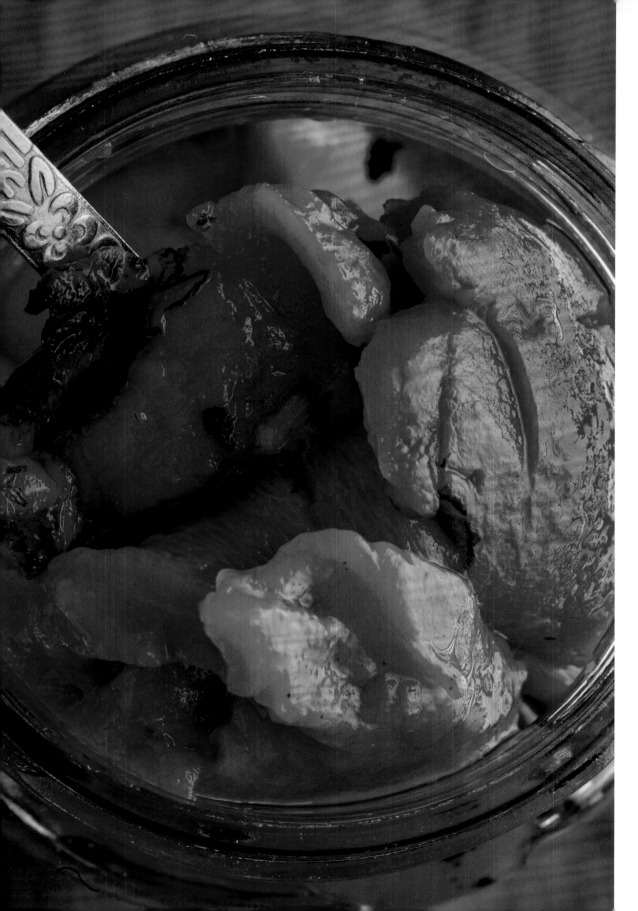

Foil-Roasted Parsnips and Carrots

Make 4 packs

Carrots and parsnips should be trimmed of their roots and stems. Scrub well to remove the soil, and peel if so desired. These foil-packs are over-the-top good when drizzled with Kale Green Onion Pesto, page 44.

Ingredients:

2 parsnips, peeled and cut into 1-inch chunks

3 carrots, peeled and cut into 1-inch chunks

1 medium onion, peeled and cut into 1-inch chunks

2 tablespoons olive oil

½ teaspoon dried thyme or dill weed

½ teaspoon kosher salt

¼ teaspoon freshly ground black pepper

Directions:

Preheat oven to 400°F. Tear four 12-inch pieces of regular-length foil.

Mix the parsnips, carrots, onion, olive oil, thyme, salt, and pepper. Portion a heaping 1 cup of vegetables into the center of a piece of foil with the long side at the top and bottom. Bring together the long sides of the foil and fold them together. Fold each end to close the packet. Repeat with remaining foil and vegetables.

Place the packets on a rimmed baking sheet and bake for 25 minutes. Allow to rest for about 5 to 10 minutes before serving.

Advantages of Foil-Roasting Vegetables

Why foil-roast a vegetable? There are many reasons. First, for portion control: you know exactly how many packets and how many people this will serve, since everyone takes one packet. Also, they are easy to grill over an indirect heat. In addition, you can prepare the packets in the morning and cook in the evening. You can even pack these in a cooler to take to a campsite or bonfire. Finally, you don't have to clean a pan! Just throw away the foil.

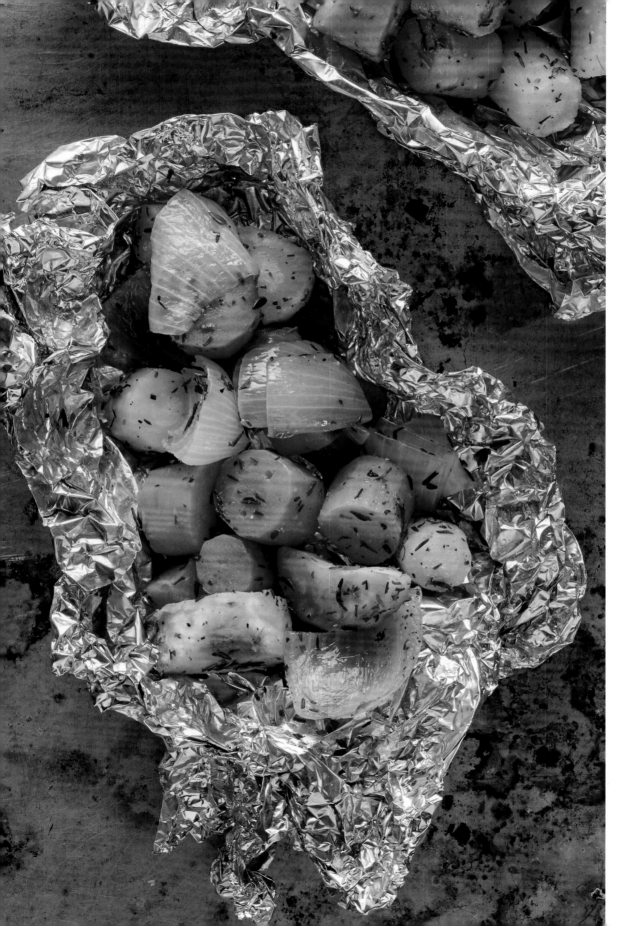

119

Suppers and Savory Bowls

With an adventurous spirit and inspiration from the pantry, you can take advantage of these recipes that include a variety of ingredients available for a plant-based supper. What makes a plant-based entree different from a side dish? Recipes for these suppers are more complex than side dishes. In addition to containing a plant-based protein of some sort, such as beans, tofu, tempeh, or lentils, these entrees can be served with a cooked whole grain or whole-grain pasta to create a complete meal. At that point, all you may need is a simple, leafy green salad to round out the meal.

Recipes

Roasted Japanese Sweet
Potatoes
  with Kale Green Onion Pesto
Fettuccine Cashew Alfredo
Barbecued Lentils
Tofu Shakshuka
Vegetable Curry with Rice
Summer Linguine
Creamy Chickpea Marinara
Cincinnati Lentil Chili
Pan-Roasted Tomato Sauce
  with Whole-Grain Penne Pasta

Curry Coconut Chickpeas
Smoky Red Beans and Rice
Kidney Bean Burgers
Moroccan Tempeh
Red Bean and Mushroom
  Jambalaya
Skillet Tofu Hash
Mushroom Ragu
Pan-Fried Tofu
Bowl Basics
Bahn Mi Bowl

Roasted Japanese Sweet Potatoes with Kale Green Onion Pesto

Serves 4

Serve this dish with hot cooked wvheat berries or brown rice. Oriental Beauty Japanese sweet potatoes have a ruby red skin and sweet, creamy interior, but you can substitute traditional sweet potatoes if Oriental Beauties are not available.

Ingredients:

1 ½ pounds Japanese sweet potato, scrubbed and cut into 1-inch chunks

6 cloves garlic, peeled

½ red onion, peeled and cut into 1-inch chunks

½ teaspoon dried thyme

½ teaspoon kosher salt

Freshly ground black pepper

2 tablespoons olive oil

Kale Green Onion Pesto, page 44

¼ cup pumpkin seeds

¼ cup dried cranberries

Directions:

Preheat oven to 425°F.

In a bowl, toss together the sweet potatoes, garlic, onion, thyme, salt, pepper, and olive oil.

Pour vegetables onto a rimmed baking sheet.

Cook for 25 to 30 minutes or until browned. Drizzle with ½ cup of pesto and toss gently to coat the potatoes with the pesto.

Spread the cooked wheat berries or rice on a large plate or small platter. Spoon the pesto-dressed potatoes on top of the cooked grain. Drizzle with more pesto if desired.

Sprinkle with pumpkin seeds and dried cranberries before serving.

Pumpkin Seeds

Pumpkin seeds are the edible seeds of pumpkin and other varieties of squash. The flat, oval seeds are light green in color. Just like any other seed, they add crunch to a dish. To preserve texture, sprinkle on top of the dish just before serving.

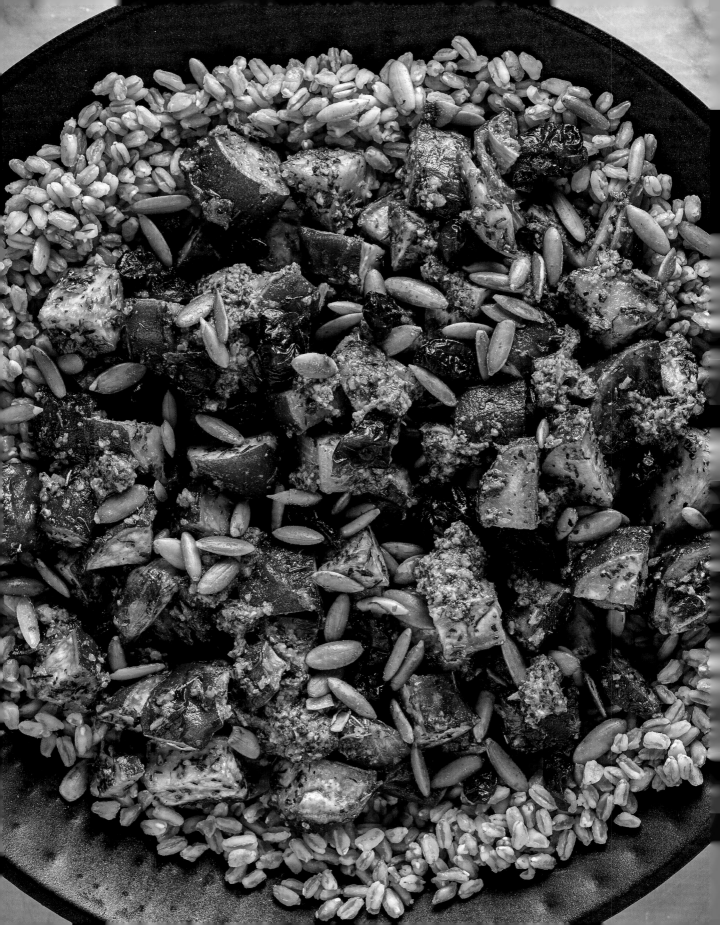

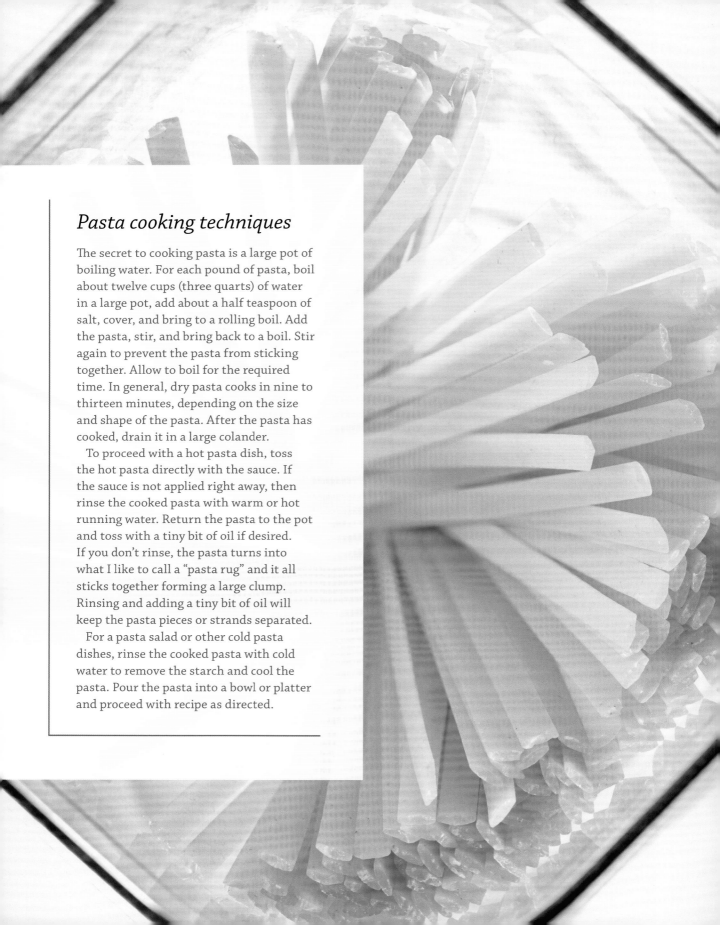

Pasta cooking techniques

The secret to cooking pasta is a large pot of boiling water. For each pound of pasta, boil about twelve cups (three quarts) of water in a large pot, add about a half teaspoon of salt, cover, and bring to a rolling boil. Add the pasta, stir, and bring back to a boil. Stir again to prevent the pasta from sticking together. Allow to boil for the required time. In general, dry pasta cooks in nine to thirteen minutes, depending on the size and shape of the pasta. After the pasta has cooked, drain it in a large colander.

To proceed with a hot pasta dish, toss the hot pasta directly with the sauce. If the sauce is not applied right away, then rinse the cooked pasta with warm or hot running water. Return the pasta to the pot and toss with a tiny bit of oil if desired. If you don't rinse, the pasta turns into what I like to call a "pasta rug" and it all sticks together forming a large clump. Rinsing and adding a tiny bit of oil will keep the pasta pieces or strands separated.

For a pasta salad or other cold pasta dishes, rinse the cooked pasta with cold water to remove the starch and cool the pasta. Pour the pasta into a bowl or platter and proceed with recipe as directed.

Fettuccine Cashew Alfredo

Serves 4 to 6

For a smooth sauce, it's essential to soak the cashews. If you plan to make this for supper, soak the cashews in the morning when you make your coffee.

Ingredients:

1 cup raw cashews

2 cups water, plus more for soaking cashews

12 ounces fettuccine

¾ teaspoon kosher salt

¼ teaspoon freshly ground black pepper

2 tablespoons olive oil

4 cloves garlic, minced

Zest of 1 lemon

1 tablespoon lemon juice (from about ½ lemon)

Optional: thinly sliced green onion

Optional: thin sliced fresh basil

Directions:

Place raw cashews in a glass or other heat-proof bowl. Cover with 1 inch hot water. Cover the bowl and soak overnight or at least 8 hours. This softens the cashews to make them easy to blend.

In a large pot of boiling water, cook fettuccine for 9 to 12 minutes until al dente or just tender to the bite. Drain in a colander and rinse with hot water.

Meanwhile, make the cream sauce while the pasta is cooking.

To make the cashew cream, drain the cashew soaking water. Using a blender mix the cashews and 2 cups water on high speed for 2 minutes. Scrape down the sides and process again until smooth and creamy. Add the salt and pepper. Process again to mix well.

In a large skillet, heat the olive oil over medium-low heat. Add the minced garlic and

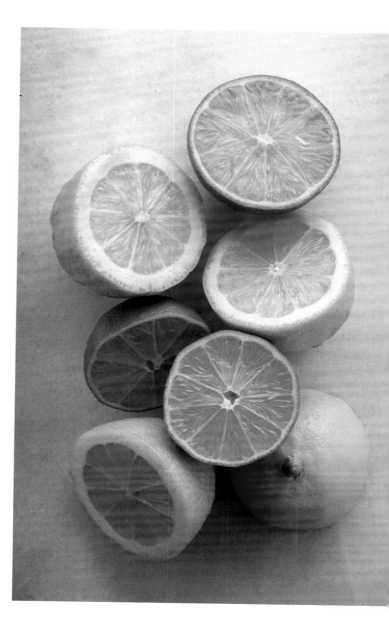

cook gently to infuse the garlic flavor into the olive oil. Strain the cashew sauce into the skillet, pouring it through a fine mesh strainer. Stir to blend well and heat until steaming. Add the cooked fettuccine a few pinches at a time using a pair of tongs or a large fork. Twist the pasta and coat it with the sauce. Mix in the lemon zest and juice. Top with chopped fresh green onion and basil if desired.

gluten free

Barbecued Lentils

Serves 4 to 6

This simple dish can be served a variety of ways—on rice or another cooked grain such as quinoa, on a toasted regular or gluten-free bun as a sloppy joe sandwich, as a topping for nachos, or as a side dish instead of baked beans.

Ingredients:

1 cup brown lentils

4 cups water

3 tablespoons olive oil

½ medium onion, chopped (about ½ cup)

3 tablespoons brown sugar

1 tablespoon apple cider vinegar

2 teaspoons chili powder

1 teaspoon smoked paprika

1 teaspoon kosher salt

½ teaspoon garlic powder

½ teaspoon onion powder

⅛ teaspoon cayenne pepper

1 cup tomato sauce

Directions:

Rinse lentils to remove any dirt and debris. Place in a large saucepan. Add water and bring lentils to a boil. Cover and reduce heat to low. Cook about 40 minutes until lentils are tender. Drain.

Meanwhile, in a large saucepan, heat the olive oil. Add the onion and cook for about 6 to 8 minutes to soften and cook the onion. Add the brown sugar, vinegar, chili powder, smoked paprika, salt, garlic powder, onion powder, and cayenne pepper to form a paste. Stir in the tomato sauce and bring to a gentle boil. Reduce heat to medium-low and let cook for 5 minutes. Add the cooked lentils and stir gently to combine with the sauce. Let cook over low heat for 5 minutes to combine well.

Buying Chopped Vegetables

Many large supermarkets showcase a large salad bar stocked with fresh, chopped vegetables. It's not always as economical for large quantities, but for small quantities of chopped vegetables such as broccoli, mushrooms, red cabbage, shredded carrot, and cauliflower, resorting to the salad bar allows you to buy only what you need, save time on prepping vegetables, and reduce waste if you have produce that spoils in your refrigerator. Many produce sections also sell packaged chopped onion, pepper, butternut squash, garlic, ginger, and herbs to save time in cooking.

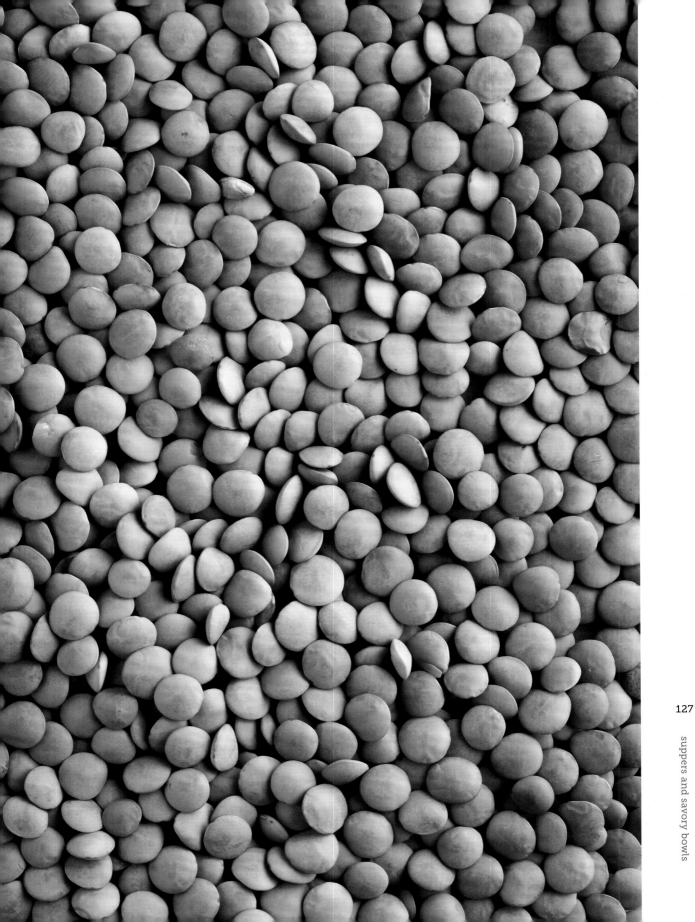

suppers and savory bowls

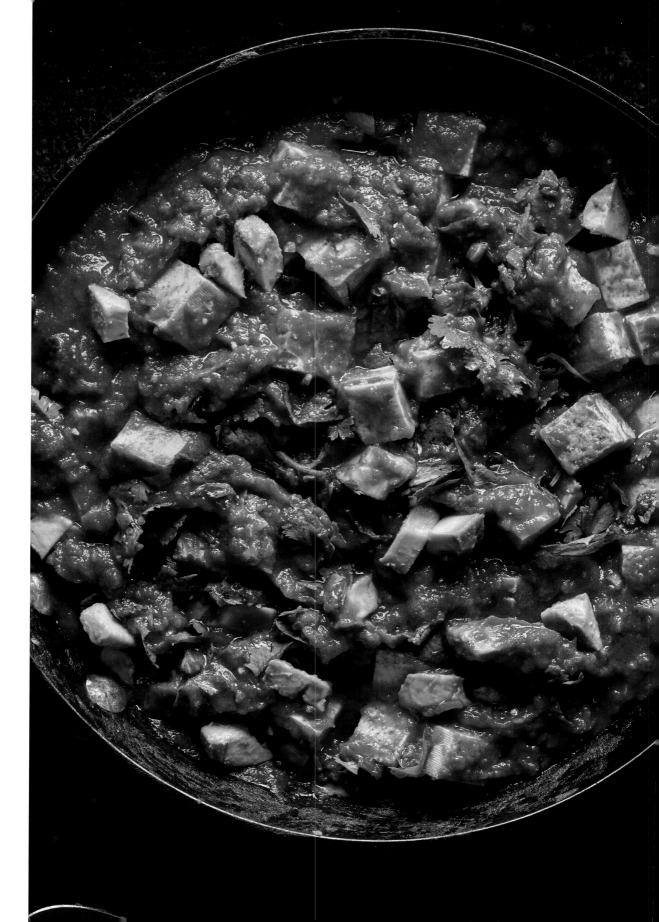

Tofu Shakshuka · gluten free

Serves 4 to 6

Even with many variations of this recipe from Spain, North Africa, and the Middle East, this dish is traditionally made with eggs (see *The Essential Pantry*, page 130). This plant-based variation substitutes extra-firm tofu for the eggs. You can use either canned green chiles or ½ cup chopped fresh Anaheim pepper. Serve over any cooked grain, or with sliced bread. I like to top this version with chopped avocado and fresh cilantro.

Ingredients:

One 14-ounce package extra-firm tofu, drained

3 tablespoons olive oil

6 cloves garlic, minced

One 4-ounce can chopped green chiles or
  1 fresh Anaheim or jalapeño pepper,
  seeded and chopped

1 teaspoon smoked paprika

1 teaspoon cumin

½ teaspoon kosher salt

One 28-ounce can crushed tomatoes

½ cup fresh cilantro

1 avocado, peeled and diced

Directions:

First, press the excess moisture out of the tofu. Slice open the tofu package and drain off the water. Place the block of tofu on a plate, and put the tofu box on top of the tofu. Fill the tofu box with heavy items, such as a 15-ounce can of beans or tomato sauce, some lemons, or apples. This places gentle pressure on the tofu and presses out excess moisture. Let the tofu sit and press for about 15 minutes.

Meanwhile, heat olive oil in a large skillet over medium heat. Add the garlic and cook for 1 minute. Stir in the green chiles, paprika, cumin, and salt. Add the crushed tomatoes and stir well.

Let simmer uncovered while you cut the tofu.

To cut the tofu into cubes, remove the tofu from the plate and place it on a cutting board. Using a paper towel, pat the excess moisture off the surface of the tofu. Slice the tofu in half (or across the middle, like a bun). You now have two rectangular slices of tofu stacked on top of each other. Cut the tofu in half widthwise (down the middle). You now have 4 sections of tofu. Cut each section into 6 cubes.

Place the tofu cubes in the tomato sauce and gently stir. Let cook for 15 minutes to heat the tofu and blend the flavors. Top with fresh cilantro and diced avocado.

Vegetable Curry with Rice

Serves 6

The coconut milk makes this curry soupy, and that's intentional. Serve over hot cooked brown or white basmati rice or any cooked whole grain, such as quinoa. The rice or other grain catches the coconut milk sauce, and the vegetables are beautiful in color and flavor.

Save the chickpea liquid to make a batch of Plant-Based Mayonnaise 1, page 48.

Ingredients:

2 tablespoons olive oil

2 teaspoons curry powder

2 teaspoons ground turmeric

½ teaspoon kosher salt

¼ teaspoon cayenne pepper

2 cups vegetable broth

One 13 ½ ounce can regular or lite coconut milk

1 head cauliflower, cut into small florets

1 sweet potato, peeled and diced

½ pound fresh or frozen whole green beans, trimmed of stem end if fresh

1 cup grape tomatoes, halved

One 15-ounce can chickpeas, drained, or 1 ½ cup cooked chickpeas

3 cups cooked basmati rice (from 1 cup uncooked)

Optional: chopped fresh cilantro

Directions:

In a large pan heat the olive oil. Add the curry powder, turmeric, salt, and pepper to create a thin paste. Slowly stir in the vegetable broth and coconut milk. Bring to a simmer. Add the cauliflower pieces and sweet potato. Bring to a low boil, and cover and cook for 10 minutes. Add the green beans, tomatoes, and chickpeas. Cook for about 12 more minutes. Serve hot over cooked basmati rice. Top with fresh cilantro if desired.

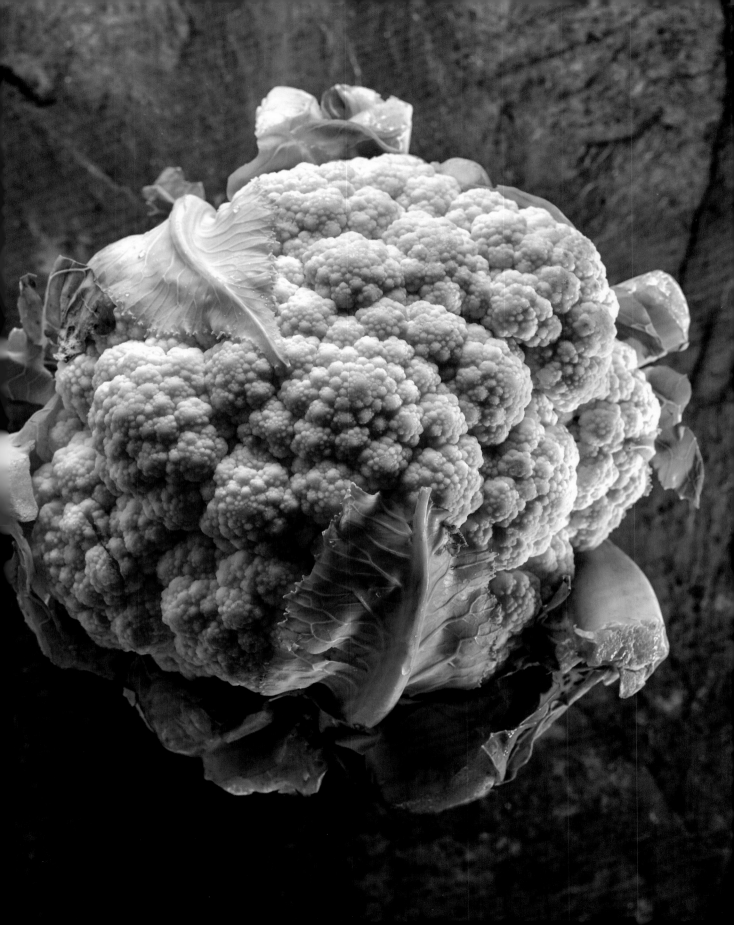

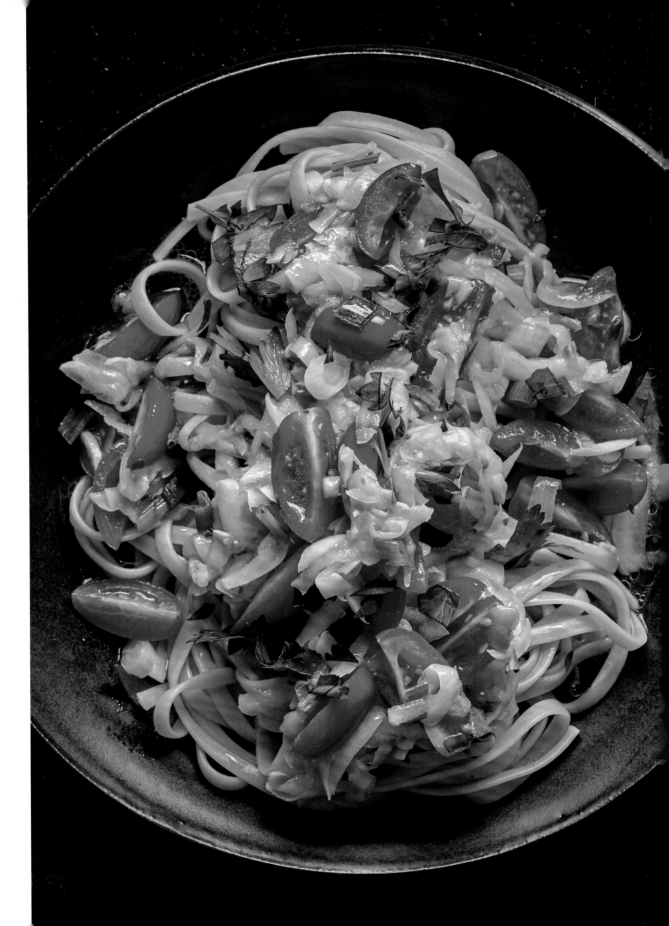

Summer Linguine

Serves 4

This summer-vegetable pasta has an olive-oil based sauce, and the ingredients shine when simply topped with fresh parsley. Reserve half a cup of pasta water before you drain the pasta, as you may need to add pasta water at the end, depending on the juiciness of the tomatoes and how much moisture is released from the squash.

Ingredients:

8 ounces linguine

½ cup olive oil, divided

6 cloves garlic, minced

¼ teaspoon red pepper flakes

4 green onions, thinly sliced

2 cups shredded yellow or zucchini squash or a combination (about 1 medium squash or 2 small squash)

1 cup grape tomatoes, quartered

½ teaspoon kosher salt

1 tablespoon lemon juice (from about ½ lemon)

¼ cup chopped fresh parsley or basil

Directions:

In a large pot of boiling water, cook the linguine for 9 to 11 minutes until al dente or just tender to the bite. Set aside ½ cup of the pasta water. Drain the pasta in a colander and rinse with hot water if there is a delay in making the sauce, or if you are cooking the pasta ahead of time. Rinsing the pasta helps prevent the pasta from sticking in a clump like a "pasta rug."

Meanwhile, in a large skillet heat ¼ cup olive oil over medium-low heat. Add the garlic and red pepper flakes and let cook for 2 minutes to flavor the oil. Increase heat to medium and add the green onion. Cook for 2 minutes. Add the squash and cook just until wilted. Stir in the quartered tomatoes, salt, and lemon juice, and additional ¼ cup olive oil and ¼ cup of pasta water if needed to thin the sauce out. Stir to blend all ingredients together. Top with chopped fresh parsley or basil.

gluten free

Creamy Chickpea Marinara

Serves 4

Raw (unroasted) cashews make the "creamy" part of this marinara sauce. Raw cashews aren't roasted or salted, and raw cashew pieces tend to be less expensive than whole raw cashews. At my supermarket, raw cashews are sold with bulk foods or in the natural food section of the store. Substitute unsalted roasted cashews if you can't find raw. Serve over cooked rice or a tube-shaped pasta, or gluten-free pasta, of your choice. Save the chickpea liquid to make a batch of Plant-Based Mayonnaise 1, page 48.

Ingredients:

½ cup raw cashews

¾ cup water, plus more for soaking cashews

2 tablespoons olive oil

3 large cloves garlic, minced

¼ teaspoon red pepper flakes

One 28-ounce can crushed tomatoes

2 tablespoons dried basil

1 tablespoon brown sugar

¾ teaspoon kosher salt

One 15-ounce can chickpeas, drained, or
   1 ½ cups cooked chickpeas

4 cups fresh baby spinach or baby kale leaves

Kosher salt

Freshly ground black pepper

Optional: chopped fresh basil

Directions:

Place raw cashews in a glass or other heat-proof bowl. Cover with 1 inch hot water. Cover the bowl and soak overnight or at least 8 hours. This softens the cashews to make them easy to blend.

After the cashews have soaked, heat oil in a large skillet with a lid over low heat. Add the garlic and red pepper flakes. Stir and cook gently for 1 minute to extract flavor. Add the crushed tomatoes, basil, sugar, and salt. Increase heat to medium-low and simmer, partially covered (to avoid splatters from tomato sauce), for 15 minutes.

Meanwhile, to make the cashew cream, drain the cashew soaking water. Using a blender mix the cashews and ¾ cup water on high speed for 2 minutes. Scrape down the blender and process again until smooth and creamy.

Strain the cashew cream into the sauce. Add the chickpeas and spinach. Simmer, partially covered, for 15 minutes to blend flavors. Season to taste with salt and freshly ground black pepper. Serve hot over your choice of cooked rice or pasta.

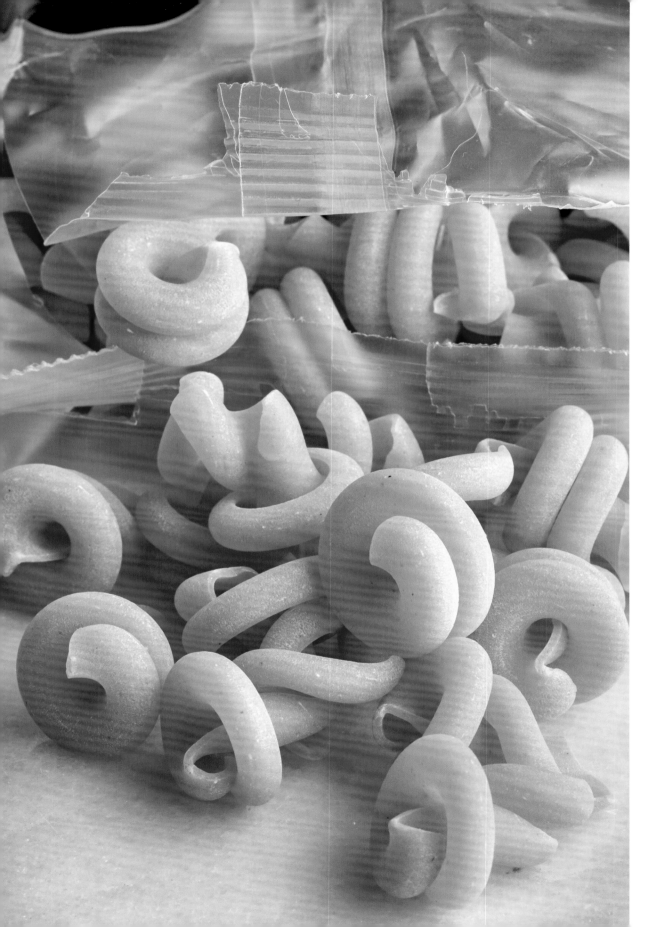

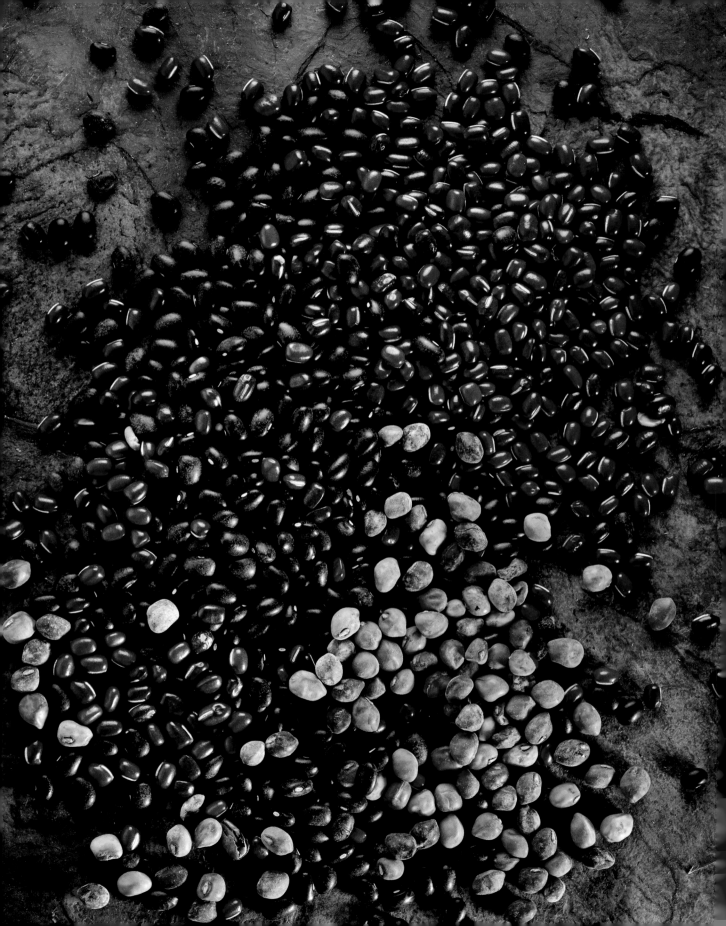

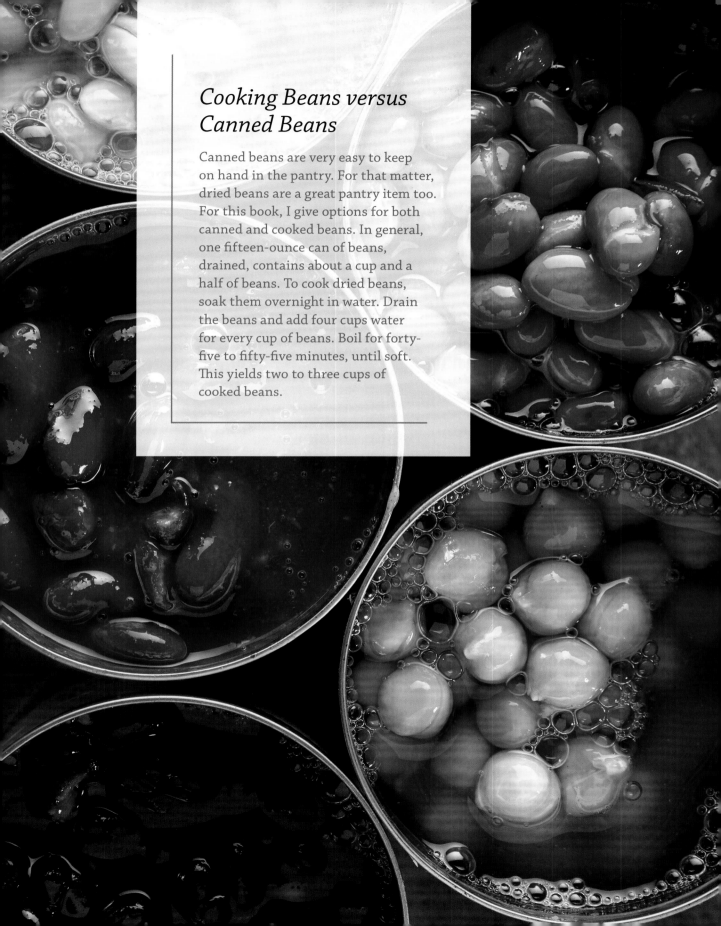

Cooking Beans versus Canned Beans

Canned beans are very easy to keep on hand in the pantry. For that matter, dried beans are a great pantry item too. For this book, I give options for both canned and cooked beans. In general, one fifteen-ounce can of beans, drained, contains about a cup and a half of beans. To cook dried beans, soak them overnight in water. Drain the beans and add four cups water for every cup of beans. Boil for forty-five to fifty-five minutes, until soft. This yields two to three cups of cooked beans.

Cincinnati Lentil Chili

Serves 6

For this recipe, use traditional brown lentils that are sold with other dried beans or in the bulk-food section of your supermarket. Serve your Cincinnati Lentil Chili as a three-way with spaghetti, chili, and avocado (where the avocado replaces the traditional cheese), or a four-way with spaghetti, chili, onion, and avocado. Hot sauce is always optional. For a 100 percent plant-based meal, serve the lentils on spaghetti squash. Oyster crackers are always welcome on the side.

Ingredients:

2 tablespoon olive oil

1 medium onion, finely chopped (about 1 cup)

3 cloves garlic, minced

2 tablespoons brown sugar

2 tablespoons cumin

1 tablespoon smoked paprika

1 tablespoon unsweetened cocoa powder

1 tablespoon cinnamon

¼ teaspoon cayenne pepper

1 teaspoon kosher salt

One 15-ounce can fire-roasted diced
    tomatoes with their juice

One 15-ounce can tomato sauce

5 cups water

¾ cup lentils

One 15-ounce can red beans, drained,
    or 1 ½ cups cooked red beans

12 ounces spaghetti

Optional toppings:

Frank's RedHot sauce

chopped avocado

finely diced onion

Directions:

In a soup pot or Dutch oven, heat the olive oil over medium-low heat. Add the onion and cook for about 6 minutes or until starting to brown. Add the garlic, brown sugar, cumin, smoked paprika, cocoa powder, cinnamon, cayenne pepper, and salt. Cook for about 1 minute until the garlic is softened and fragrant. Add the tomato, tomato sauce, water, lentils, and red beans. Bring to a simmer and cook, uncovered, over low heat for about 55 minutes or until the lentils are soft and the chili thickened.

Cook spaghetti in a large pot of boiling water. Drain and rinse with hot water.

Serve the chili sauce over hot cooked spaghetti topped with optional ingredients.

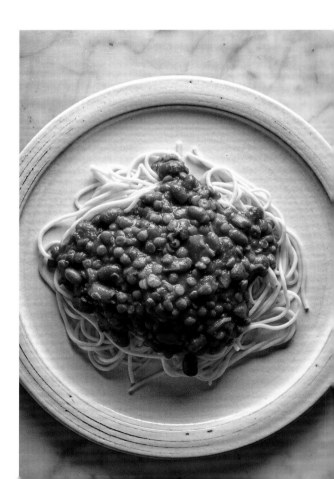

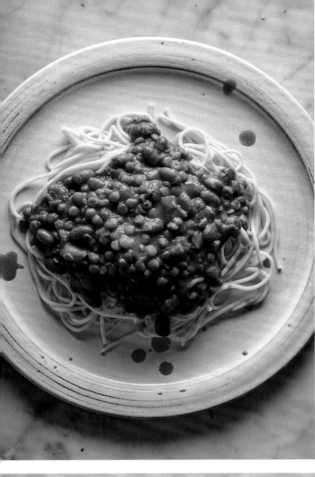
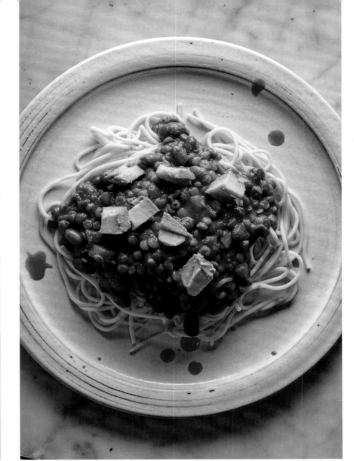
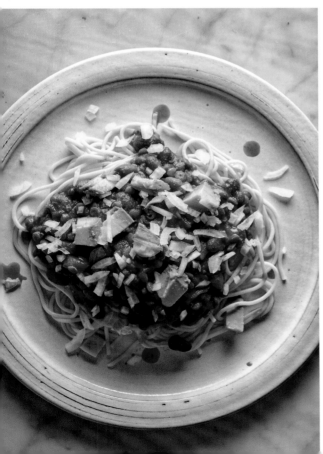
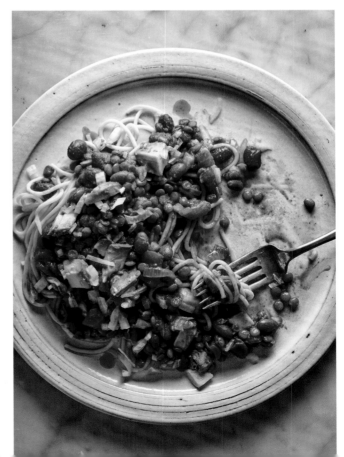

Pan-Roasted Tomato Sauce with Whole-Grain Penne Pasta

Serves 6

Grape or cherry tomatoes roasted whole in a hot skillet form the base for this fresh skillet sauce. The secret is to cook the tomatoes without disturbing them to allow the tomatoes to brown and blister. You want to keep an eye on them so they don't burn. Adjust the heat accordingly, but resist the temptation to stir the tomatoes while they initially cook. Set aside one cup of hot pasta water to adjust the consistency of the sauce as needed at the end of cooking, because the juiciness of tomatoes varies from location to location and season to season. You can use four cups of any chopped vegetables such as spinach, zucchini, or bell peppers in place of the broccoli if desired.

Ingredients:

8 ounces whole-grain penne pasta

2 tablespoons olive oil

1 pint grape tomatoes

4 cloves garlic, peeled and chopped

½ teaspoon dried thyme

½ teaspoon kosher salt

Pinch red pepper flakes

4 cups chopped broccoli (from about 1 ½ to 2-pound bunch of broccoli)

Optional: ½ cup sliced fresh basil

1 cup pasta water

Directions:

In a large pot of boiling water, cook penne for 10 to 12 minutes until al dente or just tender to the bite. Set aside 1 cup of the pasta water. Drain pasta in a colander and rinse with hot water if there is a delay in making the sauce, or if you are cooking the pasta ahead of time. Rinsing the pasta helps prevent "pasta rug."

In a large skillet, heat 2 tablespoons olive oil over medium-high heat. Add the grape tomatoes (carefully, the oil may splatter). Cover skillet and let cook for 8 to 10 minutes or until the tomatoes are blistered and browned.

When the tomatoes are cooked mash them with a wooden spoon or fork to break them open. Add the garlic, thyme, salt, and red pepper flakes. Let cook for 5 minutes to reduce and thicken the sauce.

Stir in the chopped broccoli and cover. Let broccoli cook for 3 to 4 minutes.

Stir in ¼ to ½ cup of the pasta water if needed to adjust the consistency of the sauce. Season to taste with more salt and pepper. Add the penne pasta and sliced basil, and stir well to coat the pasta in the sauce.

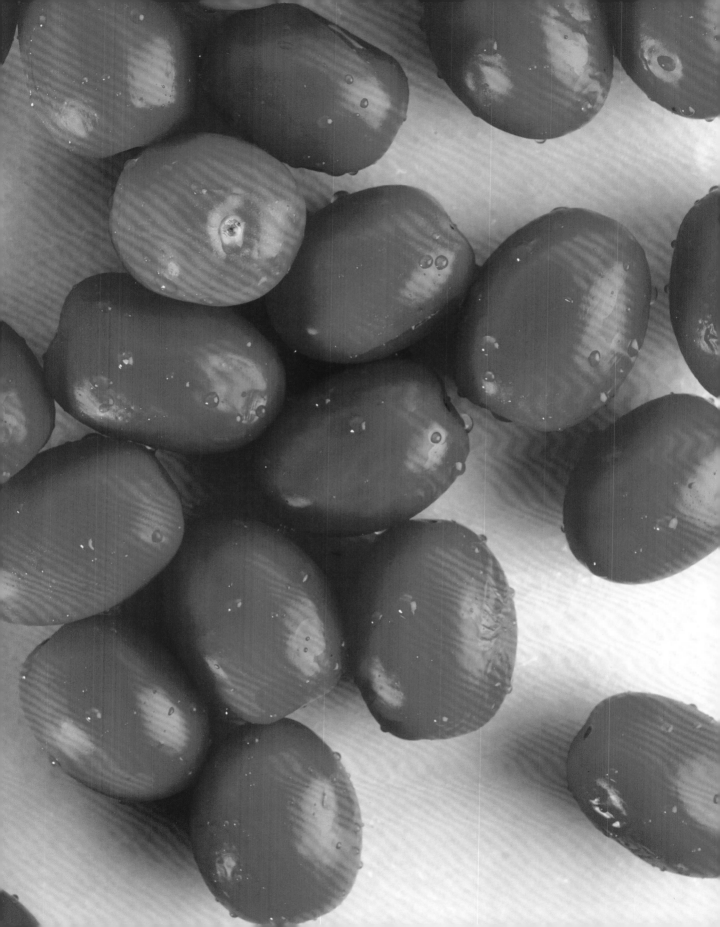

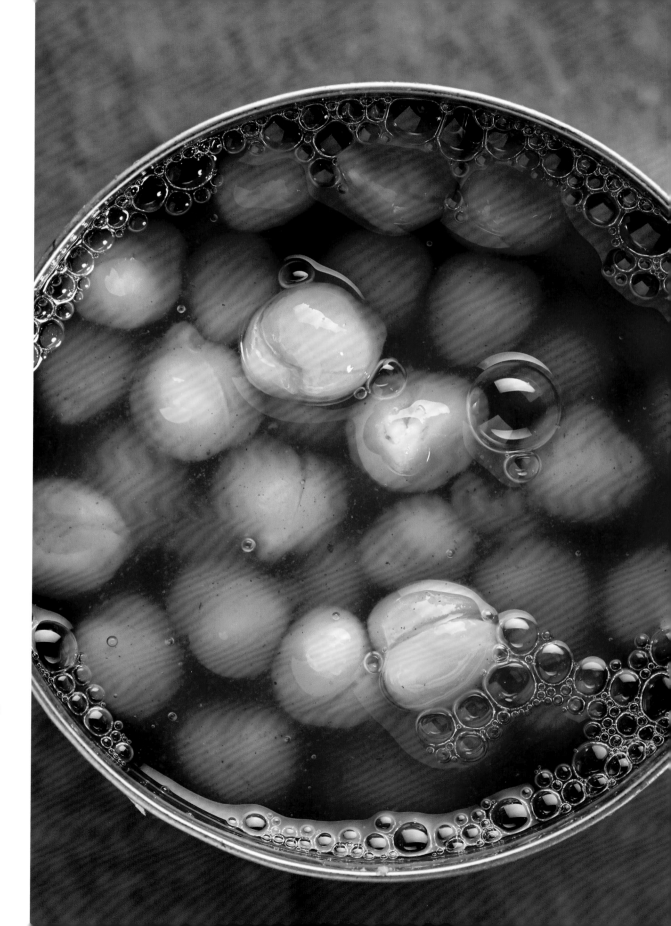

the essential plant-based pantry

Curry Coconut Chickpeas

Serves 4 to 6

Serve with hot brown rice, pita bread, and a dollop of creamy plain yogurt. Save chickpea liquid to make a batch of Plant-Based Mayonnaise 1, page 48.

Ingredients:

2 tablespoons olive oil

1 medium onion, finely chopped

2 teaspoons coriander

1 ½ teaspoon ground turmeric

1 teaspoon cumin

¼ teaspoon powdered ginger

¼ teaspoon cinnamon

⅛ teaspoon cayenne pepper

½ teaspoon kosher salt

½ teaspoon freshly ground black pepper

Two 15-ounce cans chickpeas, drained,
   or 3 cups cooked chickpeas

One 13 ½ ounce can regular or
   lite coconut milk

½ cup minced fresh cilantro

Directions:

In a large skillet, heat the olive oil over medium heat. Add the onion and cook for 6 to 8 minutes until golden and softened. Measure out the spices while the onion is cooking and mix together in a small bowl. Add the spices to the skillet and mix well with the onion. Add the chickpeas and coconut milk and stir well. Let simmer for 15 minutes. Stir in the fresh cilantro just before serving.

gluten free

Smoky Red Beans and Rice

Serves 6

Simple and quick to prepare, this bean dish is best served over cooked rice.

Ingredients:

2 tablespoons olive oil

1 medium onion, peeled and diced

2 ribs celery, sliced

1 teaspoon dried thyme

2 teaspoons smoked paprika

½ teaspoon kosher salt

Freshly ground black pepper

Two 15-ounce cans red beans, drained and rinsed, or 3 cups cooked red beans

One 15-ounce fire-roasted diced tomatoes

1 cup water

3 cups cooked rice (from 1 cup uncooked)

Optional: sliced green onion

Directions:

In a skillet, heat the olive oil over medium heat. Stir in the onion and celery and cook until both are softened, about 10 minutes. Stir in the thyme, smoked paprika, salt, and pepper and combine well. Stir in the red beans, tomatoes, and water. Stir and let cook for 15 minutes to thicken the sauce in the beans. Serve over cooked rice and top with sliced green onion.

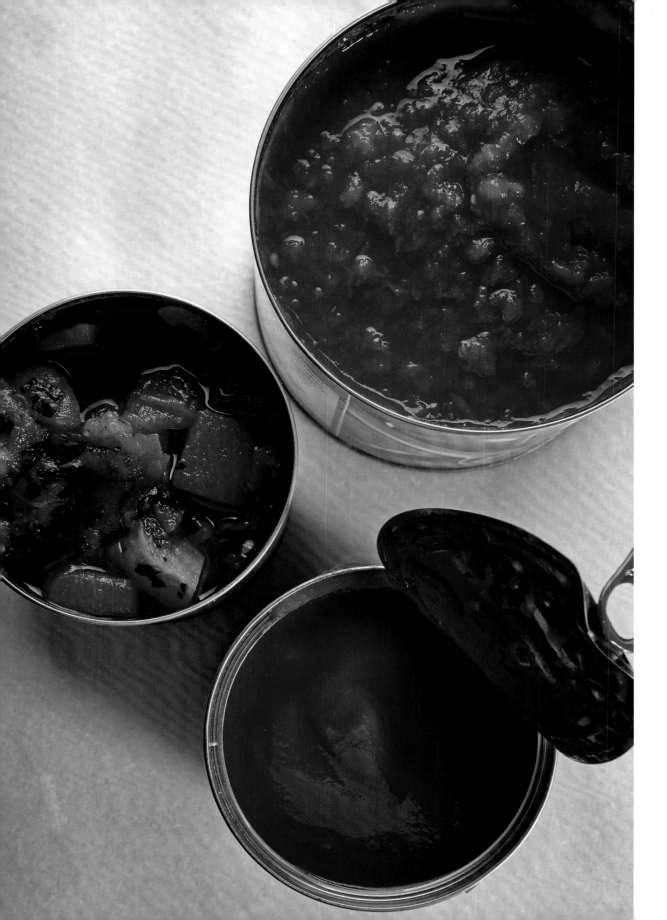

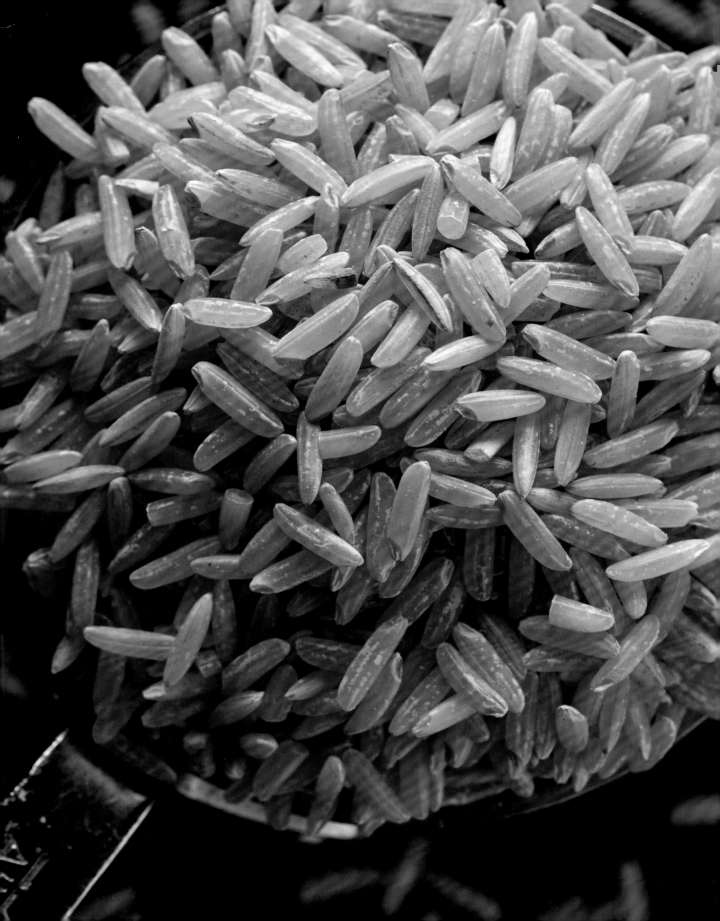

Cooking Rice

With a saucepan that has a tight-fitting lid, both white and brown rice can be cooked on the stovetop at a fraction of the cost of instant rice and instant rice mixes. The basic rule of rice is 1, 2, 3—1 cup uncooked rice, plus 2 cups of water, yields 3 cups of cooked rice. Two basic rules are to not lift the lid during cooking and not stir the rice during cooking. If you follow rule one, don't lift the lid, then rule two, don't stir, is impossible to break.

To cook rice, combine the uncooked rice and water in a saucepan. Bring to a boil over medium heat. Stir, cover, and reduce the heat to low and let cook for fifteen minutes for white rice and about forty-five minutes for long-grain brown rice. Turn off the heat and let, covered, sit for five minutes. Fluff with a fork before serving.

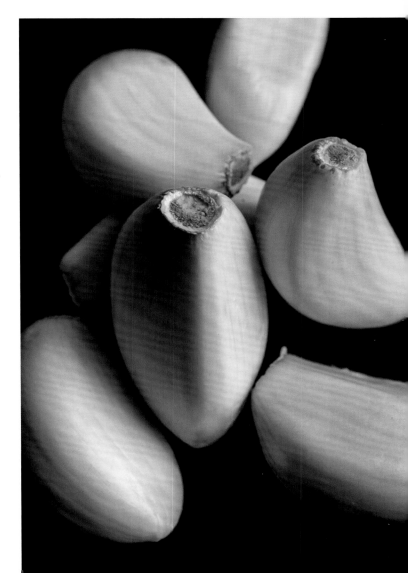

Peeled Garlic Cloves

Fresh garlic makes all the difference in a recipe. Of course, nothing is as flavorful as fresh cloves from a bulb of garlic. It stores well and you can peel and use what you need when you cook. But, in a pinch, well-stocked supermarkets may sell jars or bags of peeled garlic cloves. This saves the step of peeling garlic, and it allows you to quickly mince or crush the cloves and add fresh garlic to your recipes when needed.

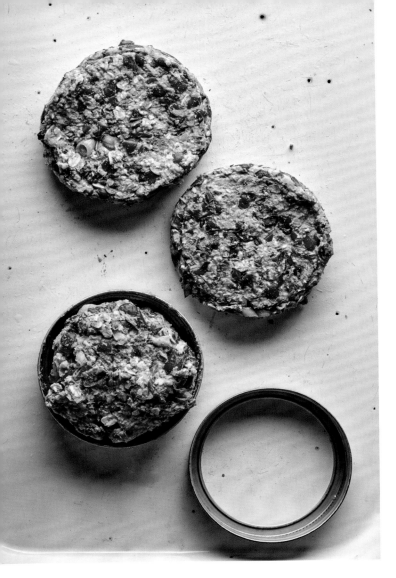

when shaping to form a patty. To shape a three-inch burger, I like to use the ring from the top of a quart-sized canning jar. Cook the burgers in a skillet, as described here, or grill them. If you do decide to grill them, be sure that the grill is well seasoned or oiled so that the burgers don't stick to the grill.

Ingredients:

One 15-ounce can kidney or red beans, drained, or 1 ½ cups cooked kidney or red beans

¼ cup thinly sliced green onion (from about 1 to 2 green onions)

½ cup finely chopped walnuts

¼ cup old-fashioned oats

¼ cup chopped fresh parsley

1 teaspoon smoked paprika

¾ teaspoon kosher salt

Freshly ground black pepper

Canola oil

Directions:

Spray a 3-inch ring from a canning jar or a round biscuit cutter with nonstick spray. Place the ring face up on a piece of parchment paper or aluminum foil.

Place the drained kidney beans in a bowl. Add the green onion, walnuts, oats, parsley, smoked paprika, salt, and pepper. Use your hands, or a mixer with the paddle attachment, to mash the beans and ingredients together until the mixture is well combined. The mixture will form a large ball. It will feel sticky but should hold together well. Divide the mixture into three equal-size portions. Shape each portion into a 3-inch patty.

In a skillet, heat a very thin layer of oil over medium heat. Add the patties and cook for 6 minutes on the first side until nicely browned. Flip the patties and reduce the heat to medium-low. Continue to cook for about 4 to 5 more minutes until browned on the other side. Keep warm until served. Dress like a burger with lettuce, tomato, and avocado if desired.

Kidney Bean Burgers

Serves 3

When testing many recipes for veggie burgers, it bothered me if I had to cook an ingredient to make the burger. So, with that in mind, I set out to create a veggie burger that doesn't require you to cook any grains or vegetables ahead of time, provided that you use canned kidney or red beans. The secret to a good veggie burger is to not have the mixture either too wet or too dry, so drain the beans well. The mixture will be sticky and stick to your hands when shaped but shouldn't be too wet. Use nice, even pressure

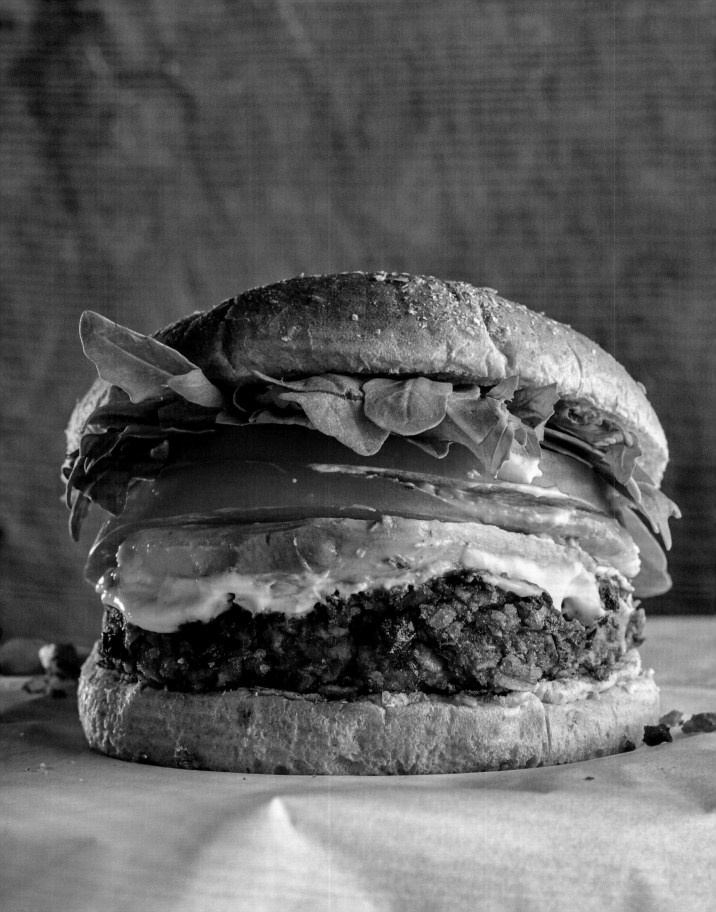

Moroccan Tempeh

Serves 3 to 4

Ingredients:

Tempeh pairs well with sturdy, highly spiced sauces such as this harissa-inspired red pepper and tomato sauce. Harissa is a flavor base used in stews and curries or as a condiment in North Africa. You can substitute cubed tofu, sautéed eggplant cubes, or cooked whole mushrooms for the tempeh if desired.

One 8-ounce package tempeh,
   cut into thin slices

1 cup vegetable broth

2 cups roasted red pepper strips

6 cloves garlic, minced

One 15-ounce can fire-roasted diced
   tomatoes, drained

1 tablespoon smoked paprika

1 teaspoon cumin

1 teaspoon coriander

½ teaspoon red pepper flakes

¼ cup olive oil

½ teaspoon kosher salt

½ teaspoon freshly ground black pepper

½ cup chopped flat-leaf parsley

½ cup golden raisins

Optional: ¼ cup pumpkin seeds

Cooked rice, barley, or wheat berries

Directions:

In a small saucepan, heat the tempeh and vegetable broth over medium heat until simmering. Cover and cook tempeh for 10 minutes. Drain the tempeh. Return the tempeh to the saucepan.

In a food processor or blender, combine the roasted red pepper, garlic, tomatoes, paprika, cumin, coriander, red pepper flakes, olive oil, salt, and pepper. Pulse to make a smooth paste.

Add the pureed red pepper paste to the tempeh mixture. Let cook for 10 minutes to heat the sauce. Top with chopped parsley, golden raisins, and pumpkin seeds. Serve with cooked rice, barley, or wheat berries to soak up the sauce.

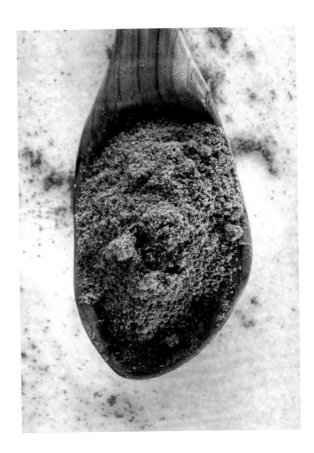

150

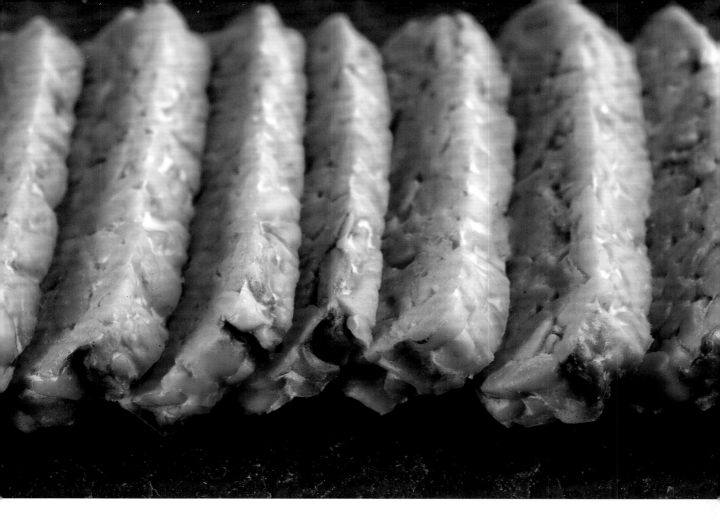

Tempeh

A flat-cake of fermented cooked soybeans, tempeh is sold in the refrigerated section of the natural or "organic" section of a supermarket. Check the sell-by date on the package and use while fresh. When cooked, tempeh holds it shape and absorbs flavors from sauces and seasonings. Uncooked, tempeh can be stored in the refrigerator for up to ten days. Tempeh can also be stored in the freezer for longer storage.

151

Red Bean and Mushroom Jambalaya

Serves 6

Jambalaya is a traditional rice-based dish, similar to Spanish chicken and rice. This recipe utilizes a dry roux to thicken the jambalaya instead of a roux made with oil and flour. The browned flour, or dry roux, has to be watched and stirred, but that's easy to do while you prepare the rest of the vegetables. When the flour is close to a peanut butter color, you mix it with vegetable broth and then stir the flour and broth mixture into the jambalaya. It will quickly thicken.

Ingredients:

½ cup brown rice

1 cup water

½ cup all-purpose flour

2 tablespoons olive oil

1 medium onion, peeled and chopped

1 green or red bell pepper, seeded and chopped

4 cloves garlic, peeled and minced

3 ribs celery, chopped

8 ounces sliced mushrooms

1 teaspoon smoked paprika

1 teaspoon dried thyme

1 teaspoon kosher salt

¼ teaspoon cayenne pepper

One 15-ounce can red beans, drained

One 15-ounce can fire-roasted diced tomatoes

2 cups vegetable broth

Hot sauce

Directions:

Combine the uncooked rice and water in a saucepan. Bring to a boil over medium heat. Stir, cover, and reduce the heat to low and let cook for 45 minutes. Turn off the heat and let sit for 5 minutes before opening the pan. Fluff with a fork.

In a skillet, brown the all-purpose flour over medium-low heat. Stir the flour frequently for about for about 25 minutes to turn the flour a brown color the shade of peanut butter. As soon as the flour has reached this color, remove it from the skillet into a bowl to stop the cooking and prevent burning. The flour is now ready for use in the jambalaya.

Meanwhile, in a Dutch oven heat the olive oil over medium heat. Add the onion, green pepper, celery, and garlic. Cook for about 8 minutes until onion and other vegetables are softened. Add the mushrooms and cook for about 6 minutes until the mushrooms release their juice. Stir in the paprika, thyme, salt, and cayenne pepper to coat all the vegetables. Add the red beans and tomatoes. Stir and heat for about 5 minutes.

Whisk the vegetable broth into the browned flour until it forms a smooth paste. Pour the flour paste into the bean and mushroom mixture. Bring to a gentle boil over medium heat. Add the cooked brown rice and serve with hot sauce.

Skillet Tofu Hash

Serves 4

A nice alternative to an omelet for breakfast, or the perfect entree for a casual supper.

Ingredients:

¼ cup olive oil

1 medium onion, peeled and diced

1 red pepper, cored, seeded and diced

2 medium red or gold potatoes, diced (about 2 cups)

1 medium zucchini, diced (about 2 cups)

½ teaspoon kosher salt

¼ teaspoon freshly ground black pepper

1 cup diced extra-firm tofu

2 green onions, thinly sliced

Optional: sriracha or hot sauce

Directions:

Preheat oven to 400°F.

In a heavy skillet or cast-iron skillet, heat the olive oil over medium heat. Add the onion, red pepper, potatoes, and zucchini. Season with salt and pepper. Cook, stirring for about 10 to 12 minutes until the onion and red pepper soften and the vegetables start to brown.

Press down on the vegetables with the back of a spatula to compact them together as much as possible. Evenly scatter the diced tofu over the vegetables. Place the skillet in the oven and bake until the potatoes are tender about 15 to 20 minutes. After baking, sprinkle with green onions and serve with sriracha or hot sauce if desired.

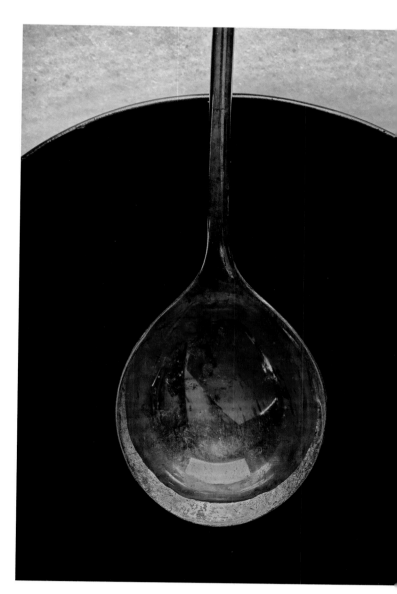

Mushroom Ragu

Serves 4

To achieve a chunky mushroom appearance, I like to buy whole button mushrooms and quarter them. Alternatively, and in the interest of saving time, sliced fresh mushrooms can be used. Serve over hot tube-shaped pasta such as penne or rigatoni, cooked rice, or a whole grain such as pearled barley or wheat berries.

Ingredients:

3 tablespoons olive oil

4 large cloves garlic, peeled and minced

16 ounces whole white button, baby bells, or crimini mushrooms, washed and quartered

1 tablespoon smoked paprika

1 teaspoon onion powder

1 teaspoon dried thyme

½ teaspoon kosher salt

⅛ teaspoon cayenne pepper

1 cup roasted red pepper strips

One 15-ounce can fire-roasted diced tomatoes

2 cups baby kale

Directions:

In a large skillet, heat the olive oil over medium heat. Add the garlic and cook over low heat until fragrant. Stir in the mushrooms and cook for about 7 minutes until they release their juice. Stir in the paprika, onion powder, thyme, salt, and cayenne pepper. Stir to coat the mushrooms. Add the roasted red pepper and tomatoes. Bring to a gentle boil and cook for 10 minutes to thicken. Add the kale and use tongs or a large fork to toss the kale with the sauce to wilt.

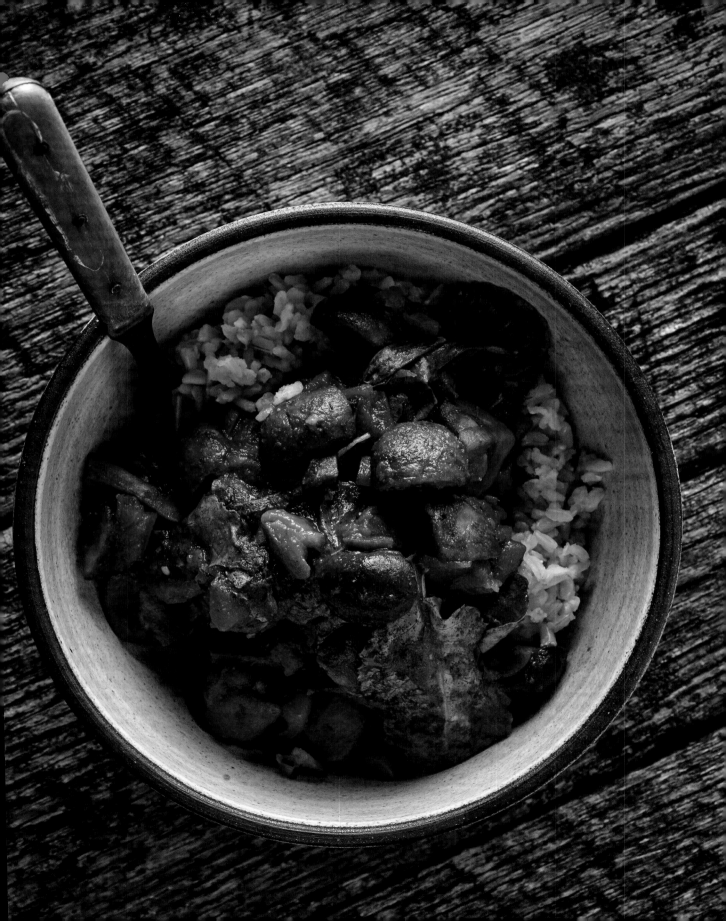

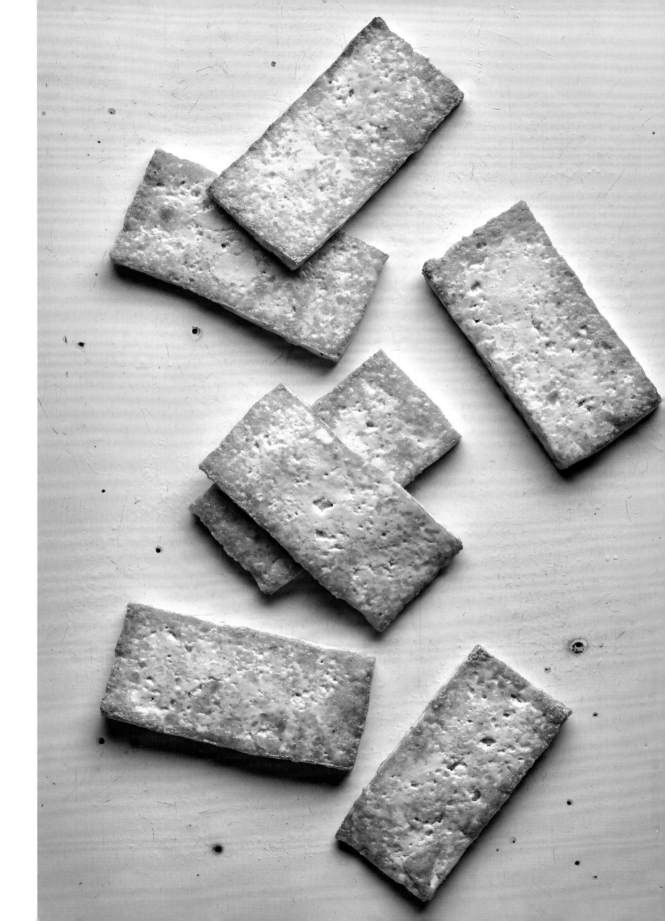

Pan-Fried Tofu

Serves 4

Planks of pressed tofu, seasoned and pan-fried, pair well with Barbecue Sauce, page 40; Tomato Curry Sauce, page 34; Spicy Marinara Sauce, page 32; or in a Bahn Mi Bowl, page 158.

Ingredients:

One 14-ounce block extra-firm tofu, drained and pressed

2 tablespoons all-purpose flour

1 teaspoon garlic powder

½ teaspoon kosher salt

¼ teaspoon freshly ground black pepper

2 tablespoons canola oil

Directions:

First, press the excess moisture out of the tofu. Slice open the tofu package and drain off the water. Place the block of tofu on a plate and put the tofu box on top of the tofu. Fill the tofu box with heavy items such as a 15-ounce can of beans or tomato sauce, some lemons, or apples. This places gentle pressure on the tofu and presses out excess moisture. Let the tofu sit and press for about 15 minutes.

Remove the box from the top of the tofu and move the tofu to a cutting board. With a paper towel, pat the excess moisture off the surface of the tofu. Slice the tofu in half across the middle. You now have two rectangular pieces of tofu. Turn each piece of tofu and cut across the short side into ½-inch thick slices. You should end up with about 16 "planks" of tofu.

In a shallow dish, mix the flour, garlic powder, salt, and pepper.

Heat the canola oil in a large skillet over medium heat. Dredge each tofu slice in the flour to coat both sides. Cook the tofu slices in batches, browning on the first side for 5 minutes. Turn the tofu and continue to cook for 3 to 4 minutes until the second side is brown and crispy. Keep warm in a 200°F oven.

Bahn Mi Bowl

Serves 1

A beautiful, fresh combination of pickled vegetables, fried tofu, and sriracha mayonnaise, this recipe recreates the Bahn Mi in a bowl. Have Spicy Refrigerator Pickles, page 18, ready.

Ingredients:

½ cup uncooked quinoa

1 cup water

½ cup Plant-Based Mayonnaise, page 48

1 tablespoon sriracha

3 pieces Pan-Fried Tofu, page 157

¼ cup fresh cilantro leaves

Spicy Refrigerator Pickles

Directions:

To prepare quinoa, place it in a fine mesh strainer. Rinse under cold water for 1 minute to remove bitterness. Place the rinsed quinoa in a small saucepan and add 1 cup water. Over medium heat, bring to a boil. Reduce heat to low and simmer, uncovered until the water is absorbed, about 10 minutes. Remove from heat and cover. Let sit for 5 minutes. Fluff with a fork and move to a plate to cool.

Meanwhile, mix mayonnaise with sriracha sauce.

In a bowl, place a layer of quinoa, top with planks of fried tofu. Top tofu with pickled vegetables, fresh cilantro, and drizzle with sriracha mayonnaise. Serve immediately.

How to Press and Drain Tofu

To press the excess moisture out of the tofu, open the tofu package and drain off the water. Place the block of tofu on a plate and put the empty tofu box on top of the tofu. Fill the tofu box with heavy items such as a fifteen-ounce can of beans or tomato sauce, some lemons, or apples. This places gentle pressure on the tofu and presses out excess moisture. Let the tofu sit and drain for about fifteen minutes. Remove the box from the top of the tofu and move the tofu to a cutting board. With a paper towel, pat the excess moisture off the surface of the tofu. Use as described in the recipe.

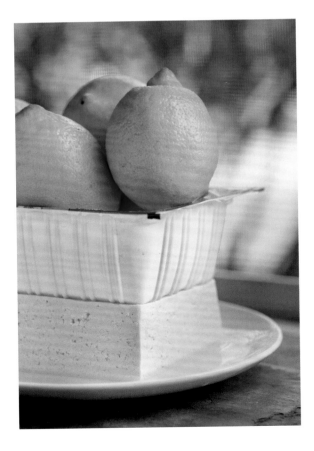

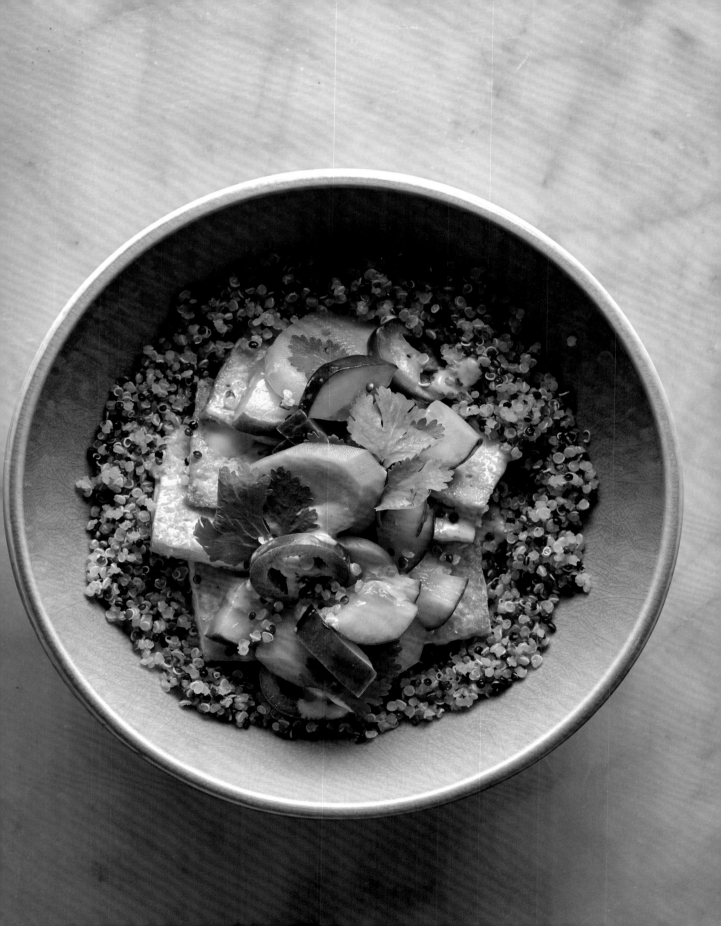

Bowl Basics

You can create your own bowls using the following guidelines.

First, layer a base on the bottom of the bowl:
Base ideas include:
Cooked brown rice
Cooked quinoa
Cooked whole-grain or other pasta
Sweet Potato and Onion Hash Browns, page 106
Spiced Rice Pilaf with Golden Raisins and
    Almonds, page 108
Mac and No Cheese, page 105

Second, add a layer of vegetables:
Refrigerator Pickles, page 18
Pickled red onion
Braised Eggplant and Lemon, page 110
Roasted Cardamom Carrots, page 114
Sesame Honey Brussels Sprouts, page 106
Edamame Succotash, page 117
Chopped fresh romaine
Massaged kale, page 85
Baby arugula
Baby spinach or spring greens

Top with a plant-based protein:
Barbecued Lentils, page 126
Pan-Fried Tofu, page 157
Kidney Bean Burger, page 148

Top with nuts:
Pumpkin seeds
Chopped walnuts

Gild the lily:
Tahini Sauce, page 47
Almond Curry Pesto, page 43
Kale Green Onion Pesto, page 44
Barbecue Sauce, page 40
Fire-Roasted Tomato Salsa, page 37
Plant-Based Mayonnaise, page 48
Jalapeño peppers
Sriracha
Diced avocado
Chopped Kalamata or green olives
Sprinkle of Chili Powder or Curry Powder,
    page 30

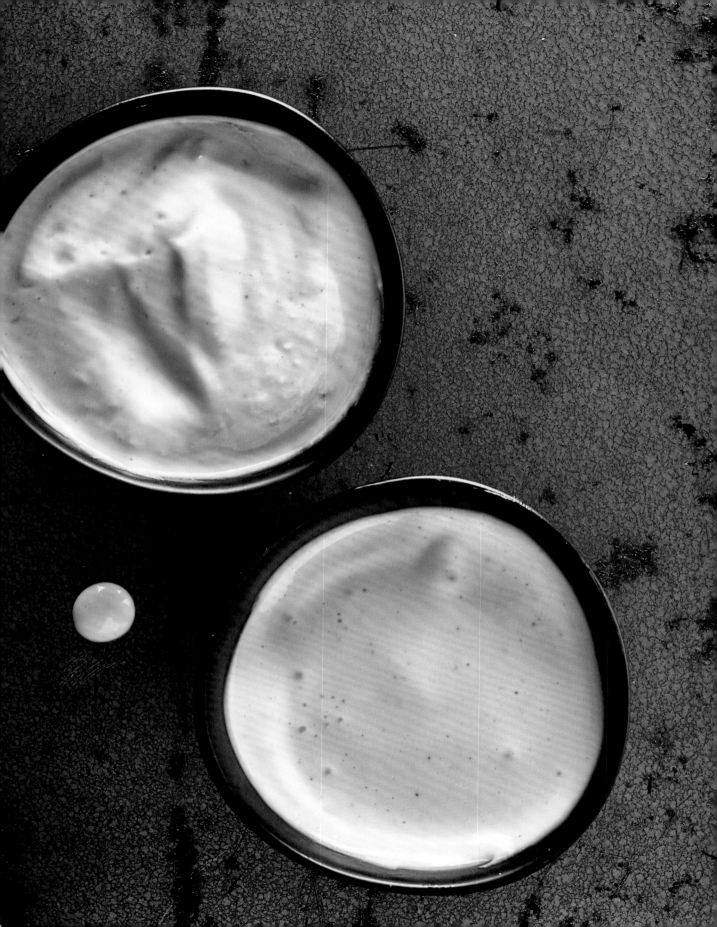

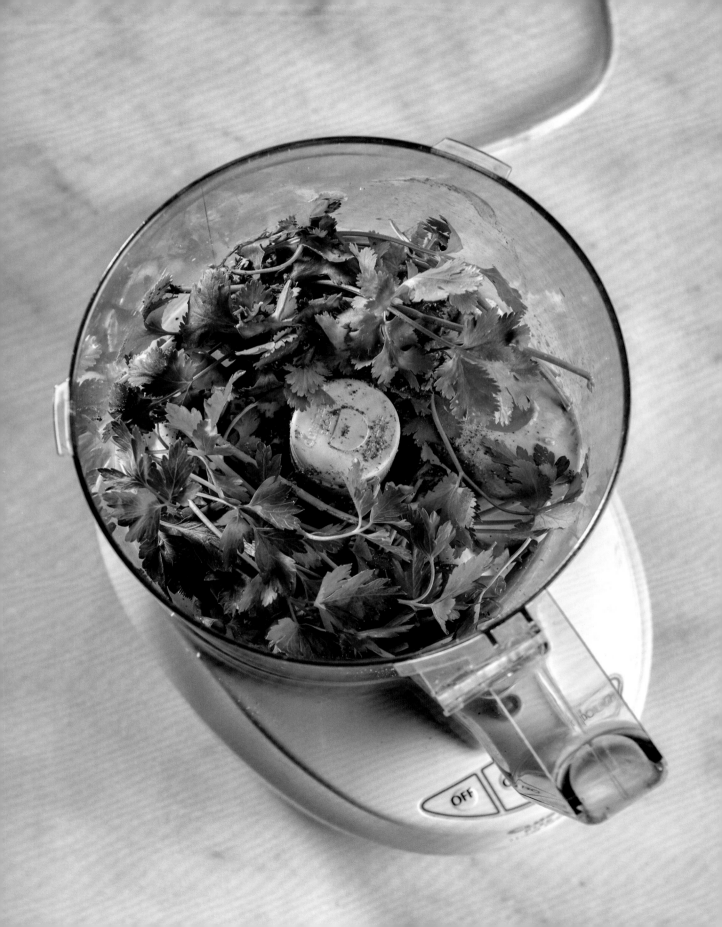

❧ Cooking Equipment List

In addition to *The Essential Plant-Based Pantry* ingredient list, a kitchen needs basic equipment to successfully prepare the recipes in this book.

Blender: Either a countertop or immersion blender works for blending soups and making cashew cream or pesto, but for crushing ice or making a smoothie, countertop models work best.

Box grater: Use this to grate your own vegetables.

Can opener: The old-fashioned hand-cranked model with the new-fangled twist mechanism doesn't leave a sharp edge. Plus it stores away in a drawer.

Cast-iron skillet: No kitchen should be without one. Take care when using and washing it so it doesn't lose its seasoning.

Colander: This tool is essential for washing fruits and berries and draining pasta.

Dutch oven: This pot is especially useful for making soups, stews, chilis, or braising vegetables. Two terrific Dutch ovens are the cast-iron version from Lodge and the enameled cast iron version from Le Cruset. Both are heavy and conduct heat slowly, but once they get hot, they retain heat beautifully.

Food processor: For certain kitchen tasks, nothing beats a food processor—mixing pizza dough and pie crust, making pesto and salsa, chopping nuts, shredding cabbage, and grating large quantities of cheese.

Garlic press: Some argue the virtues of pressed versus minced garlic, but I'm not a discerning enough cook to tell the difference in most recipes. Pressing garlic is a fast way to cut fresh garlic, so I often use a garlic press instead of mincing.

Hot mitts: I like hot mitts that extend up to the bend in my elbows. At this length, the mitts protect my hands from hot pans and my forearms from the steam when draining hot pasta and even the occasional bump on the oven rack. And unlike square pot holders or a dish towel, I can wear them like gloves, allowing me to keep a good grip on hot dishes.

Knives: There are three knives that every well-stocked kitchen should have. The chef's knife is used for slicing, chopping, and cutting. The paring knife is good for making small cuts and doing any knife work such as peeling while you are holding the vegetable or fruit "in the air" such as a potato or apple, as opposed to placing the vegetable or fruit on a cutting board and cutting it. The serrated knife is used to slice bread and tomatoes. Shop for a knife that fits your hand. Keep your knives sharp, and don't put them in the dishwasher.

Measuring cups and spoons: For measuring liquids, two- or four-cup glass models are most useful. For measuring dry ingredients and small amounts of liquids, both smaller measuring cups and measuring spoons are a must.

Oven proof baking dishes: I use primarily 13 × 9 × 2-inch and 15 × 11 × 2-inch baking dishes.

Parchment paper: Used primarily for baking, it's readily available in rolls at the supermarket.

Rimmed baking sheets: Also called half sheet pans, rimmed baking sheets have multiple uses in the kitchen. Those used for the recipes in this book are 17 1/2 × 12 1/2 × 1 inches.

Saucepan: A three- to four-quart saucepan is a nice size for soups and cooking small quantities of pasta.

Silicone spatula or cooking spoons: They used to be called rubber spatulas, but now everything is made of silicone. You can buy scrapers and spoons made from silicone, and they are good for stirring foods while cooking. Wooden spoons also work well for cooking.

Skillet: Most often I use a twelve-inch ovenproof skillet with sloped sides. My favorite brand is All-Clad. They might seem expensive at first, but if you buy the stainless-steel version, you may never have to replace it. My ten-inch cast-iron skillet is a close second favorite. I like the depth of the skillet, and because it's well-seasoned, I can cook almost anything in it, including foods with tomatoes or tomato sauces.

Strainer: A strainer with fine mesh openings comes in handy to rinse quinoa.

Tongs: I use tongs all the time to toss salads, serve long strands of pasta, and turn vegetables in a skillet or Dutch oven, or on the grill.

Whisk: For making homemade vinaigrette and salad dressings nothing beats a whisk. I like one with long, thin wires.

❧ Index

Page numbers in italics refer to photographs.

fresh, 78; tips for massaging, 85; Vegetable Kale Soup, 65

Kidney Bean Burgers, *148, 149*

kitchen basics: concept of essential plant-based pantry; equipment list, 163–164; menu suggestions, 8–9; pantry ingredients list, 6–7; pantry makeover, 8; tips for using recipes, 10

knives, 164

lemons: Apple and Celery Salad with Tahini Dressing, 96; Blueberry Lemon Quinoa Salad, 89; Braised Eggplant and Lemon, 110, *111*; Carrot Golden Raisin Salad, 90, *91*; Cashew Cream Sauce, 38; Fettucine Cashew Alfredo, 125; Green Hummus, 22; Kale Green Onion Pesto, 44, *45*; Plant-Based Mayonnaise 1, 48; Roasted White Bean Dip, 24; Spicy Marinara Sauce, 32; Summer Linguine, *132, 133*; tips for using, 10; Tomato Curry Sauce, 34; Vegan Caesar Dressing, 48; Warm White Bean Salad, 84

lentils: Barbecued, 126; Cincinnati Lentil Chili, *138, 139*; Curried Red Lentil, Quinoa, and Apple Soup, 62, *63*; Lentil Barley Soup, 66; Tortilla Soup, 74; types of, 64

lettuce, Spring Roll Salad with Sweet Chile Vinaigrette, 100

limes: Cilantro Lime Jalapeño Mayonnaise, 49; Fire-Roasted Tomato Salsa, 37; Sriracha Peanut Sauce, 55; Sweet Chile Vinaigrette, 56, 100; tips for using, 10

Linguine, Summer, *132, 133*

Mac and No Cheese, *104,* 105

Marinara, Creamy Chickpea, 134

Marinara Sauce, Spicy, 32

mayonnaise (plant-based): Cayenne Garlic, 49; Cilantro Lime Jalapeño, 49; Garlic Mayonnaise or Aioli, 49; Green Goddess, 49; Plant-Based Mayonnaise 1, 48; Plant-Based Mayonnaise 2, 48; Sriracha, 48; Tofu Eggless Salad, *82, 83*; Vegan Caesar Dressing, 48

measuring cups and spoons, 164

Mediterranean Salad, *94,* 95

menus, 8–9

Mild Sauce for Buffalo Tofu, 20

mint: Napa Cabbage Slaw with Sriracha Peanut Sauce, *92,* 93; Spring Roll Salad with Sweet Chile Vinaigrette, 100; Sweet and Spicy Curried Chickpea Salad, 80; Tomato Curry Sauce, 34; Warm White Bean Salad, 84

Moroccan Tempeh, 150

mung bean sprouts, Spring Roll Salad with Sweet Chile Vinaigrette, 100

mushrooms: Mushroom Ragu, 154, *155*; Red Bean and Mushroom Jambalaya, 152

Napa Cabbage Slaw with Sriracha Peanut Sauce, *92,* 93

nondairy milk alternatives: Banana Cocoa-Nut Smoothie, 16; Cashew Cream of Broccoli Soup, 72; Cashew Cream Sauce, 38; Turmeric Cocoa Latte, *14. See also* coconut milk

oats, Kidney Bean Burgers, *148, 149*

olives: Mediterranean Salad, *94,* 95; Olive Spread, 21

onions: Cincinnati Lentil Chili, *138, 139*; Foil-Roasted Parsnips and Carrots, 118, *119*; Skillet Tofu Hash, 153; Sweet Potato and Onion Hash Browns, 106

onions, green: Green Goddess Mayonnaise, 49; Kale Green Onion Pesto, 44, *45*; Kidney Bean Burgers, *148, 149*; Napa Cabbage Slaw with Sriracha Peanut Sauce, *92,* 93; Skillet Tofu Hash, 153; Summer Linguine, *132,* 133

onions, red: Mediterranean Salad, *94,* 95; Pickled Red Onion and Cucumber, 18; Roasted Japanese Sweet Potatoes with Kale Green Onion Pesto, 122, *123*; Roasted White Bean Dip, 24; tips for soaking, 95; Warm White Bean Salad, 84

oregano, Home-Blended Chili Powder, 30

Pan-Fried Tofu, *156,* 157

Pan-Roasted Tomato Sauce with Whole-Grain Penne Pasta, 140

pantry list, 6–7

parchment paper, 164

parsley: Almond Curry Pesto, 43; Carrot Golden Raisin Salad, 90, *91*; Fresh Herb Vinaigrette, 52, *53*; Green Goddess Mayonnaise, 49; Kidney Bean Burgers, *148, 149*; Moroccan Tempeh, 150; Napa Cabbage Slaw with Sriracha Peanut Sauce, *92,* 93; Olive Spread, 21; Summer Linguine, *132, 133*

parsnips, Foil-Roasted Parsnips and Carrots, 118, *119*

pasta: Cincinnati Lentil Chili, *138, 139*; Creamy Chickpea Marinara, 134; Fettucine Cashew Alfredo, 125; Mac and No Cheese, *104,* 105; Mushroom Ragu, 154, *155*; Pan-Roasted Tomato Sauce with Whole-Grain Penne Pasta, 140; Summer Linguine, *132, 133*; tips for cooking, 124; tips for using, 10

peanut butter: Banana Cocoa-Nut Smoothie, 16; Sriracha Peanut Sauce, 55

peppers, red or green: Bean Salad with Lime Vinaigrette, 99; Braised Eggplant and Lemon, 110, *111*; Edamame Succotash, 117; Moroccan Tempeh,

Food and nutrition expert *Maggie Green* is the owner of The Green Apron Company. The Green Apron specializes in culinary nutrition, food and nutrition writing, and recipe and cookbook development. As a professionally trained chef and registered dietitian, Green is a sought-after culinary nutrition expert and cookbook industry consultant.

Green is a registered and licensed dietitian with a degree in dietetics from the University of Kentucky. After a career in clinical dietetics and food service management, Green opened The Green Apron Company. Following her work as a personal chef for over one hunded clients in the greater Cincinnati area, Green successfully transitioned to the publishing industry.

As a cookbook editor, Green edited American's favorite cookbook the *Joy of Cooking* (2006) as well as *BakeWise* (2008), by Shirley Corriher. As a food and nutrition writer, Green's experience includes writing for Humana's Active Outlook Program and as ghost writer for recipe chapters in health and nutrition books. As an author, Green wrote her first cookbook, *The Kentucky Fresh Cookbook*, in 2011. *The Kentucky Fresh Cookbook* explores seasonal cooking and regional foods of Kentucky. In 2016, Green wrote her second cookbook, *Tasting Kentucky: Favorite Recipes from the Bluegrass State. Tasting Kentucky* showcases one hundred recipes from restaurants and inns all across the state of Kentucky. In 2015, Green launched Cookbook Camp, which offers virtual individual and group coaching programs for aspiring cookbook authors. Green is a member of the Academy of Nutrition and Dietetics as well as the International Association of Culinary Professionals.

Green lives in Ft. Wright, Kentucky, with her husband, the best male cook she knows, and a shaggy dog also named Maggie. They have three children who all enjoy sharing time in the kitchen and around the table.

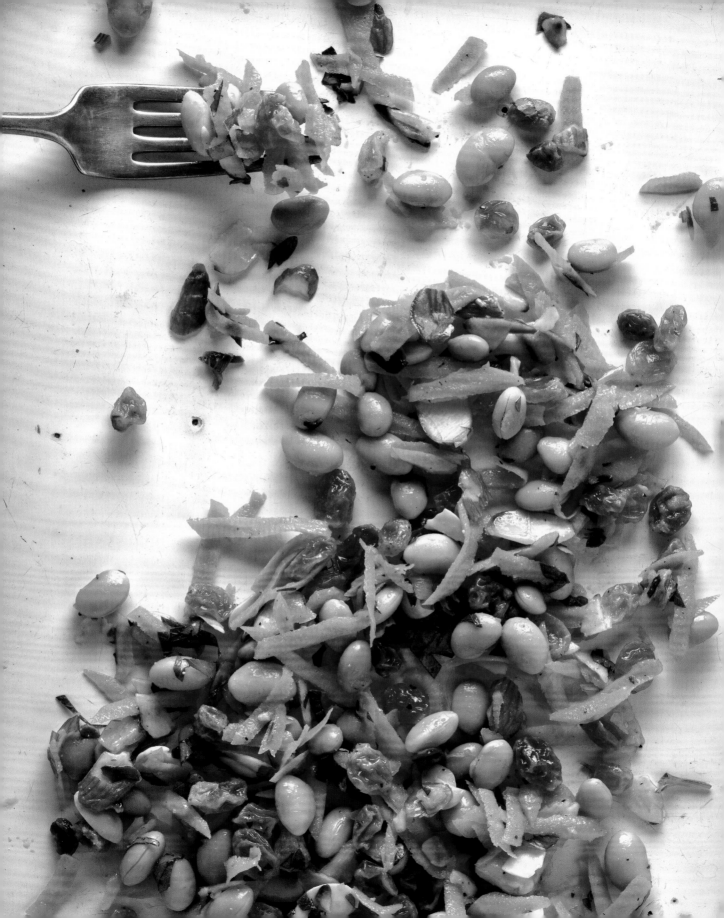